Higher FRCS

Higher FRCS: SBAs for Section 1 of the General Surgery FRCS Examination is designed to help prepare for the first part of the Fellowship of the Royal Colleges of Surgeons (FRCS) general surgery exam. Due to a lack of preparatory resources for the exam, this book intends to bridge the gap, offering updated guidelines and information which will help candidates succeed in their exam. It acts as a supportive revision guide that will enrich other FRCS exam resources.

This book aims to provide an updated approach to the FRCS exam. Using questions written by practicing surgeons, the book will offer more contemporary revision materials, touching on topics not widely covered in other FRCS revision materials. Readers will gain familiarity with the style of the FRCS exam as *Higher FRCS* uses a style reflective of the exam to enhance the candidate's knowledge, confidence, and preparation.

The audience for this book includes general surgery trainees who are preparing for their higher exams (including FRCS), alongside surgical trainees taking the MRCS. It is also a beneficial resource for students in other medical courses studying for surgical exams.

Higher FRCS

SBAs for Section 1 of the General Surgery FRCS Examination

Edited by

Muhammad Rafay Sameem Siddiqui

Associate Editors

Mohamed Baguneid
Arnab Bhowmick
Jemma Bhoday

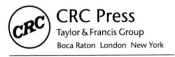

CRC Press
Taylor & Francis Group
Boca Raton London New York

CRC Press is an imprint of the
Taylor & Francis Group, an **informa** business

First edition published 2023
by CRC Press
6000 Broken Sound Parkway NW, Suite 300, Boca Raton, FL 33487-2742

and by CRC Press
4 Park Square, Milton Park, Abingdon, Oxon, OX14 4RN

CRC Press is an imprint of Taylor & Francis Group, LLC

© 2023 Taylor & Francis Group, LLC

Library of Congress Cataloging-in-Publication Data
Names: Siddiqui, Muhammad Rafay Sameem, editor. | Baguneid, Mohamed, editor. | Bhowmick, Arnab, editor.
Title: Higher FRCS : SBAs for section 1 of the general surgery FRCS examination / edited by Muhammad Rafay Sameem Siddiqui ; associate editors M. Baguneid, A. Bhowmick, J. Bhoday.
Description: First edition. | Boca Raton, FL : CRC Press, 2023. |
Includes bibliographical references and index.
Identifiers: LCCN 2022036246 (print) | LCCN 2022036247 (ebook) | ISBN 9781032117263 (hbk) | ISBN 9781032076126 (pbk) | ISBN 9781003221234 (ebk)
Subjects: LCSH: Surgery–Examinations, questions, etc. | Surgery–Examinations–Study guides.
Classification: LCC RD37.2 .H54 2023 (print) | LCC RD37.2 (ebook) | DDC 617.0076–dc23/eng/20220929
LC record available at https://lccn.loc.gov/2022036246
LC ebook record available at https://lccn.loc.gov/2022036247

ISBN: 9781032117263 (hbk)
ISBN: 9781032076126 (pbk)
ISBN: 9781003221234 (ebk)

DOI: 10.1201/9781003221234

Typeset in Times
by codeMantra

To The One, Habib, Bushra, Aaliyah-Noor,
Huda, my parents and sisters.

Contents

Preface

Hope and fear are 2 wings of the same bird (Proverb)

The proverb above so eloquently describes the extremities of human emotion during the final period of our training. A culmination of years of hard work which could result in futility is real, and the fear is fuelled by stories of those rarities (thankfully only rarities) that do not make it and end up somewhere else – often lost and unable to pick themselves up from this glorious defeat, that is, the surgical training pathway. The bells of 'imposter syndrome' toll exacerbating a somewhat irrational fear of being 'found out'. Also, there is a fear of looking into the eyes of our loved ones to tell them that we have failed. It is a nauseating effect, something that I have personally experienced after finding out that I needed to take the part 1 exam for a second time. Nothing prepares you for that moment.

However, there is hope: a hope that the revision has been worthwhile, that the 2 weeks, 3 months or 12 months have been enough to get you through one of the final hurdles before becoming a consultant, that you can finally be settled with a single permanent job and that you never have to do another exam again!

It is upon these emotions that this book was conceptualised and ultimately delivered. It is a concern that the lives of excellent trainees like ourselves are placed on hold. We hope that through our collective experience, no one will need to sit the exam twice.

The purpose of any book or question bank is to facilitate our revision. No single resource is going to be exhaustive.

We have, however, looked at the syllabus for general surgery and have covered as much of it as possible. One of the biggest challenges many of us found before the exam was that the questions in the exam were not truly reflected in any of the revision resources. This led to a lot of frustration, and a group of us wanted to make sure that after we finished, we would create a resource that would seem more similar to the exam.

This book is the result of these efforts, and I hope that it will lead you to success in your first or subsequent attempts.

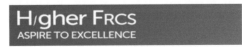

Section 1 of the FRCS is one of the hardest exams you will take. Sometimes it is too overwhelming, and you just does not know where to start or whom to ask.

Higher FRCS offers a wide range of resources from starter courses to viva practice.

On purchasing this book, you are eligible to take advantage of a 15% discount on the online question bank at www.higherfrcs.co.uk, offering you an additional 1100 questions to revise.

Our further resources include the following:

A STARTER COURSE

https://www.eventbrite.co.uk/e/frcs-section-1-tips-and-techniques-tickets-158506554371

We will talk you through how to start, practice questions and talk about technique and application. The feedback received so far has been excellent and has helped candidates save that initial revision time searching for resources and identifying the approach to the exam.

We cover the following aspects during the course

1. Introduction to the exam
2. The syllabus
3. Timings of the exam
4. How to start and revise
5. Timetabling
6. Revision Resources
7. Exam question practice
8. Identifying keywords
9. Overview of cancer pathway protocols to help you start.

A LAST MINUTE VIVA COURSE

https://www.eventbrite.co.uk/e/higher-frcs-viva-practice-registration-335851489847

Everyone is happy to help but when it comes down to it, bosses often have limited time. They may not be up to date with the latest exam format, and it all leads to anxiety. Practice with us and get tailored feedback specifically for you.

There will be a maximum of five participants being vivaed, so these sessions are far more focussed towards you as an individual candidate.

This will observe candidates to help identify weaker areas and areas for feedback to hone in on things before the exam.

Each candidate is vivaed in general, with sub-specialty and academic sections totalling 60 minutes of dedicated viva practice with feedback.

SOCIAL MEDIA

We have an incredible social media presence on Twitter, Instagram and Facebook. We post regular free MCQs and also hold support sessions immediately before and after the exam.

- Twitter handle @HFrcs
- Instagram handle @h_frcs
- Facebook Page www.facebook.com/HigherFRCS/
- Facebook Group www.facebook.com/groups/4904996052860240
- We are with you every step of the way!

DISCOUNT CODE

Code for Online Question Bank

- www.higherfrcs.co.uk
- Enter Code: HFRCS2023

Editors

Muhammad Rafay Sameem Siddiqui, South Tyneside and Sunderland Royal Hospitals NHS Trust. Muhammad Siddiqui is a consultant in colorectal surgery who trained in South West London and Exeter. He graduated from Liverpool University and completed his PhD in MRI assessment of rectal cancers at Croydon University Hospital, The Royal Marsden Hospital and Imperial College.

He passed his FRCS in 2020 and understands the challenges and difficulties related to the exam. Due to a discrepancy between the FRCS exam and the resources available, Siddiqui dedicated a period of time to developing a resource to help plug that gap.

Mohamed Baguneid has been a consultant vascular and endovascular surgeon for over 15 years. He has held many senior clinical leadership roles in the NHS and more recently in the government healthcare system in the United Arab Emirates. His leadership roles have focussed on clinical strategy and service transformation. He is passionate about setting up and delivering educational programmes and is one of the co-founders and organisers of the Alpine FRCS General Surgery Course.

Arnab Bhowmick MBChB FRCSEd (Gen Surg) is a Consultant Colorectal and General Surgeon at Lancashire Teaching Hospitals Trust. Appointed as a consultant in 2006, he has been a leader in undergraduate education and post-graduate surgical education. He co-founded the highly successful Alpine FRCS course, for which he has been an organiser and senior faculty member for 16 years. He is also a viva examiner on the ACPGBI Advanced Coloproctology Course.

Jemma Bhoday is a post-CCT fellow in colorectal surgery at Frimley Park Hospital. She graduated from St George's Medical School, London, in 2006 and completed her surgical training in SW London. She passed her FRCS in 2020.

Contributors

Sarah Abdelbar
South Tyneside & Sunderland
Royal Hospitals NHS Trust
Sunderland, United Kingdom

Sulaiman Saif Salim Alshamsi
Chair of Vascular Surgery
Consultant Vascular and Endovascular
Surgeon
Tawam Hospital
Al Ain, United Arab Emirates

Mohamed Baguneid
Consultant Vascular Surgeon
SEHA
Abu Dhabi, United Arab Emirates

Ajay Belgaumkar
Consultant Surgeon in Upper
Gastrointestinal and General
Surgery
Surrey and Sussex Healthcare NHS
Trust
Redhill, United Kingdom

Arnab Bhowmick
Department of Colorectal Surgery
Royal Preston Hospital
Preston, Lancashire, England

Simon Chang-Hao Tsao
Breast & Endocrine Surgeon
Royal Australasian College of
Surgeons, Senior Lecturer (Hon)
University of Melbourne
Melbourne, Australia

John Corson
Consultant General & Colorectal
Surgeon
South Tyneside & Sunderland Royal
Hospitals NHS Trust
Sunderland, United Kingdom

Michael Courtney
Consultant Upper GI Surgeon
South Tyneside & Sunderland
Royal Hospitals NHS Trust
Sunderland, United Kingdom

Paul C. Dent
Consultant General, Endocrine &
Thyroid Surgeon
Croydon University Hospital
Thornton Heath, United Kingdom

Hazim Eltyeb
Surgical Registrar
South Tyneside & Sunderland
Royal Hospitals NHS Trust
Sunderland, United Kingdom

Muhammad Fahim
Speciality Registrar
Surrey and Sussex Healthcare NHS
Trust
Redhill, United Kingdom

Golam Farook
Consultant Colorectal & General
Surgeon
South Tyneside & Sunderland
Royal Hospitals NHS Trust
Sunderland, United Kingdom

Ioannis Gerogiannis
Consultant Emergency Surgeon
Kingston Hospital NHS Trust
Kingston, United Kingdom

Petrut Gogalniceanu
Consultant Transplant & Vascular
    Access Surgeon
Guy's & St. Thomas NHS Foundation
    Trust
London, United Kingdom

Stephen Holtham
Consultant General & Colorectal
    Surgeon
South Tyneside & Sunderland
    Royal Hospitals NHS Trust
Sunderland, United Kingdom

Tanvir Hossain
Trauma Fellow
Nottingham University Hospitals
Nottingham, United Kingdom

Mike Kipling
Consultant Colorectal & General
    Surgeon
South Tyneside & Sunderland
    Royal Hospitals NHS Trust
Sunderland, United Kingdom

Kaushal Kundalia
Senior Clinical Fellow
Guy's & St. Thomas NHS Foundation
    Trust
London, United Kingdom

Nabeel Merali
Research Fellow
Minimal Access Therapy Training
    Unit (MATTU) Research
    Department
Royal Surrey Hospital NHS
    Foundation Trust
Guildford, United Kingdom

Brendan J. Moran
Consultant Surgeon, Peritoneal
    Malignancy Institute, Basingstoke
Hampshire Hospital NHS Foundation
    Trust
Basingstoke, United Kingdom

Osama Moussa
Post-CCT Fellow in Upper GI Surgery
    and Bariatrics
Ashford and St. Peter's Hospitals NHS
    Trust
Stanwell, United Kingdom

Aya Musbahi
Senior Upper GI Surgical Registrar
South Tyneside and Sunderland
    Royal Hospitals NHS Trust
Sunderland, United Kingdom

Hamed Noor Khan
Consultant Breast & General Surgeon
University Hospitals Coventry &
    Warwickshire
Coventry, United Kingdom

Carol Norman
Consultant Oncoplastic Breast
    Surgeon
Croydon University Hospitals
    Royal Hospitals NHS Trust
Thornton Heath, United Kingdom

Rachel O'Connell
Consultant Oncoplastic Breast
    Surgeon
The Royal Marsden NHS Foundation
    Trust
Sutton, United Kingdom

Hussien Rabee
Consultant Vascular Surgeon
Smart Center, Countess of Chester
    Hospital
Chester, United Kingdom

Kumaran Ratnasingham
Consultant in Upper GI Surgery and
   Bariatrics
Ashford and St. Peter's Hospitals NHS
   Trust
Stanwell, United Kingdom

James Royle
Consultant Colorectal & General
   Surgeon
South Tyneside & Sunderland
   Royal Hospitals NHS Trust
Sunderland, United Kingdom

Mitesh Sharma
Bariatric Fellow
South Tyneside & Sunderland
   Royal Hospitals NHS Trust
Sunderland, United Kingdom

Jigna Sheth
Consultant Paediatric and Neonatal
   Surgeon
Royal Alexandra Children's Hospital,
   University Hospitals Sussex
Sussex, United Kingdom

Yuen Soon
Head and Senior Consultant Upper GI
   Surgery
Ng Teng Fong General Hospital
   National University Health System
Jurong East, Singapore

Kiran Sran
Consultant Transplant & Vascular
   Access Surgeon
Guy's & St. Thomas NHS Foundation
   Trust
London, United Kingdom

Irena Stefanova
General Surgery Registrar
Frimley Health NHS Foundation Trust
Frimley, United Kingdom

Christophe Thomas
Surgical Registrar
South Tyneside & Sunderland
   Royal Hospitals NHS Trust
Sunderland, United Kingdom

Alexios Tzivanakis
Consultant Surgeon, Peritoneal
   Malignancy Institute, Basingstoke
Hampshire Hospital NHS Foundation
   Trust
Basingstoke, United Kingdom

Peter Vaughan-Shaw
Post-CCT Fellow Robotic Surgery
South Tyneside & Sunderland
   Royal Hospitals NHS Trust
Sunderland, United Kingdom

Nicholas T. Ventham
Post-CCT Fellow Robotic Surgery
South Tyneside & Sunderland
   Royal Hospitals NHS Trust
Sunderland, United Kingdom

Introduction

The FRCS is probably one of the most difficult exams you will do. Part of the challenge lies in the stage of life you are at and juggling family, friends, work and the need to operate. It is really important that all of those around you are on board with what you are trying to achieve and understand the pressures on you to attain those objectives.

The exam is also quite expensive and stands at around £2,000 which needs to be paid upfront and is something you may wish to start saving for over a period of 12 months if you do not have it spare at the moment.

A good way to approach this is by starting early typically 3–6 months before the exam and really doing your best. Do not use an attempt as a trial because you only have four attempts, and they go really quickly.

Another great way of maximising your time is by creating a thorough timetable factoring in your personal and work time as well, identifying dead time such as waiting for the computer to load or walking from one ward to another. I would also recommend getting a group together for moral support during the journey and having sessions where you discuss questions that you are not quite sure about. The JCIE has some sample questions that are useful but dissimilar to the exam, so be mindful of that. You can access them at this link:

https://www.jcie.org.uk/Utils/DocumentGenerator.aspx?Type=CMS&docID =1fd94c07-5220-4ebb-bbc2-8de6c31e8492

Everyone revises slightly differently, so you have to have insight into the best way that you work. In terms of revision, we would certainly recommend you start with an area that is familiar to you because psychologically it will help and motivate you during this period of study. Have a particular deadline for finishing the area that you know well and then move to more challenging areas that you are not familiar with, commonly transplant and skin.

You may have heard a lot of people talk about marginal gains when referencing the exam, and this is very true. Often people will fail by 1 mark and that can be really gutting. A recount or reassessment of your paper usually does not lead anywhere and is expensive. Furthermore, the final positive outcome is that you void your attempt rather than have your marks changed which makes the process less than worthwhile unless you are on your last attempt. Make sure that when you create your timetable, every area is covered on the syllabus, and this will maximise your chances for success.

Do not forget local and regional teaching days.

The local and regional teaching days are designed to target deficiencies in knowledge and are very useful. It can be tricky when it clashes with clinical work but they are designed for you and some regions also have FRCS teaching days as part of regional teaching. The Association of Surgeons of Great Britain and

Ireland (ASGBI) is recently looking into developing a nationwide teaching programme that brings local hospital teaching to a global audience and is certainly something to look out for.

Each of these resources has its benefits and pitfalls. We would encourage you to use all of these resources to give you the maximum chances of success as they enhance your revision in slightly different ways and in different circumstances.

We really hope everyone passes.

Good luck!

1 Bariatric Surgery

Kumaran Ratnasingham and Osama Moussa

Q1. A 49-year-old diabetic male patient has a BMI of 48 kg/m^2 and is on the Tier 3 programme for weight management. During his surgical consultation, the patient declares he has had previous surgery. Which surgery precludes the possibility of a Roux-en-Y gastric bypass?
   A. Laparotomy for peritonitis
   B. Open cholecystectomy
   C. Ileocaecal resection for Crohn's disease
   D. Previous gastric band
   E. Hiatal hernia surgery

Q2. A 68-year-old female Asian patient presented to the emergency department with significant right-sided abdominal pain, fevers and rigours. Further assessment discovered deranged inflammatory markers, bilirubin and liver enzymes. She underwent a laparoscopic single-anastomosis bypass surgery 2 years prior, and currently, her BMI is 40 kg/mB. An ultrasound reported gallstones with evident cholecystitis and a dilated common bile duct (CBD) of 12 mm. Which of the below is the next mode of management?
   A. ERCP (endoscopic retrograde cholangiopancreaticography)
   B. Percutaneous transhepatic percutaneous CBD cannulation
   C. Laparoscopic-assisted trans-gastric ERCP
   D. Laparoscopic bile duct exploration
   E. MRCP

Q3. A 49-year-old Asian patient completes the Tier 3 weight management programme for 9 months and now has a BMI of 30.9 kg/m^2. She has a background of diabetes, hypertension, hiatus hernia and Barrett's oesophagus. As a bariatric surgical consultant, what is the best way to manage this patient after appropriate MDT discussion?
   A. Laparoscopic sleeve gastrectomy
   B. Continue Tier 3 management for 3 more months
   C. Discharge as the patient no longer qualifies for Tier 4 surgery
   D. Single anastomosis bypass
   E. Roux-en-Y gastric bypass

Q4. A 32-year-old lady presents to your emergency department with an inability to tolerate solids or fluids orally. During the consultation, she reveals that she had a laparoscopic gastric band in the private sector 9 months ago. She seems very anxious, tachycardic and dehydrated. What is your initial step in management?
   A. Serum blood and lactate
   B. Abdominal X-ray
   C. IV fluids and purine
   D. CTAP with oral contrast
   E. Emergency deflation of the band

DOI: 10.1201/9781003221234-1

Q5. A 34-year-old female patient, with a BMI of 51 kg/m² who has diet-controlled diabetes attends your bariatric clinic for the first time. She is unsure which bariatric procedure is best for her. She asks you which is the most common bariatric procedure worldwide.
   A.   Gastric band
   B.   SADI
   C.   Laparoscopic sleeve gastrectomy
   D.   Roux-en-Y gastric bypass
   E.   Single anastomosis gastric bypass

Q6. Which of the below patients does not qualify for Tier 4 bariatric surgery after 6 months on the Tier 3 weight management programme?
   A.   A 37-year-old female with a BMI of 38 kg/m² with no comorbidities
   B.   A 42-year-old Persian female with a BMI of 31.7 kg/m² and new-onset diabetes
   C.   A 29-year-old female with a BMI of 40 kg/m², diabetic and hypertensive, with a past history of bulimic eating tendencies
   D.   A 42-year-old male with a BMI of 52 kg/m² with severe obstructive sleep apnoea (OSA) and is currently a smoker
   E.   A 52-year-old male with a BMI of 48 kg/m² and Barrett's oesophagus

Q7. A 49-year-old patient presents 6 months after a Roux-en-Y Gastric Bypass (RYGB) with colicky abdominal pain and intermittent vomiting. After a radiological diagnosis, a laparoscopy confirmed an internal hernia. Up-to-date evidence confirmed that the closure of defects significantly reduces the risk of internal hernias. However, it increases the incidence of re-operation for which of the following?
   A.   Colonic injury
   B.   Port site hernia
   C.   Mesenteric haematoma
   D.   Non-specific abdominal pain
   E.   Twisting at the jejuno-jejunostomy

Q8. A 60-year-old Asian male patient is investigated 18 months post-Roux-en-Y gastric bypass for epigastric pain and vomiting and is found to have a marginal anastomotic ulcer. Despite prolonged treatment, a follow-up endoscopy reported a non-healing ulcer. What would you be suspicious of?
   A.   Patient continuing to smoke
   B.   Resistant *Helicobacter pylori*
   C.   Underlying micro-leak and collection at the anastomosis
   D.   Alcohol abuse
   E.   Gastro-gastric fistula

Q9. A 35-year-old Caucasian female with a BMI of 37 kg/m² presents at 11 months after one anastomosis gastric bypass with burning feet sensation and signs of peripheral neuropathy. The most common micronutrient associated with neurological symptoms is
   A.   Iron
   B.   Selenium

    C. Vitamin D
    D. Vitamin B1
    E. Copper

Q10. A 35-year-old female patient attends a follow-up clinic 6 months after a sleeve gastrectomy. She informs you that she no longer consumes alcohol but suffers significant reflux and is unable to lie flat at night. An endoscopy reports grade III oesophagitis and gastric erosions but no strictures. She asks about management options available; what is the most reasonable management?
    A. Long-term high-dose proton pump inhibitor (PPI)
    B. Laparoscopic fundoplication
    C. Laparoscopic sero-myotomy
    D. Roux-en-Y gastric bypass
    E. Single anastomosis gastric bypass

Q11. Evidence reports several mechanisms for weight loss; what is the most favourable postoperative physiological cause of greatest weight loss?
    A. Metabolic surgery increases the number of gut peptide-expressing enteroendocrine cells
    B. Faster delivery to distal ileum post malabsorptive surgery stimulates enteroendocrine cells to release satiety hormones
    C. Faster gastric emptying
    D. Vagal afferents terminating at the nucleus tractus solitarius
    E. GLP-1 slow gastric emptying

Q12. A 32-year-old female with a BMI of 49 kg/m² attends her first appointment for consideration of bariatric surgery. She is very motivated for surgery and has achieved all the multidisciplinary criteria. She asks you what is the most likely physiological mechanism responsible for comorbidity resolution. Which of the following is not associated with resolutions of comorbidities post-bariatric surgery?
    A. Gut hormones
    B. Bile acid kinetics
    C. Changes in behaviours and weight management
    D. Functional improvement
    E. Rapid gastric emptying

Q13. Bariatric surgery in adolescents is recommended in all of the criteria given below except:
    A. A 17-year-old with a BMI of 42 kg/m² with OSA
    B. An 18-year-old female patient with class 2 obesity who underwent 9 months of supervised weight loss under a paediatric weight loss clinic
    C. A male adolescent showing commitment to medical and psychological postoperative treatment
    D. A 16-year-old with a BMI of 38.9 kg/m²
    E. An adolescent with an eating disorder and a BMI of 46 kg/m²

Q14. A 49-year-old female patient attends the pre-operative assessment clinic prior to a Roux-en-Y gastric bypass. She is very concerned when she is made aware of the morbidity and mortality risks. Which of the following pre-operative factors is NOT associated with a reduction in postoperative complications:
A. A BMI of 51 kg/m^2
B. Three-week liver shrinkage diet
C. A 5% pre-operative weight loss
D. CPAP compliance in OSA
E. Pre-operative glycaemic optimisation

Q15. What is the most validated tool used to ascertain risk stratification and stratify patients' suitability for surgery:
A. King's Obesity Staging Score
B. Eastern Cooperative Oncology Group (ECOG) performance status
C. Edmonton Obesity Staging Score
D. The American Society of Anaesthesiologists (ASA) physical status classification
E. Obesity Surgery Mortality Risk Score (OSMRS)

Q16. A 49-year-old Asian male patient who has a BMI of 51 kg/m^2 is a type 2 diabetic. Which of the following criteria is not an indication for surgery?
A. Fasting glucose of <6.1 mmol/L
B. Long-standing poorly controlled diabetes despite all medical efforts
C. HbA1C of 9.1%
D. Adequate fasting glucose and HbA1c control with advanced nephropathy
E. HbA1C of 7.8% with retinopathy

Q17. A 29-year-old patient with a BMI of 48 kg/m^2 attends a bariatric clinic and enquires about pregnancy and childbearing. Why is pregnancy contraindicated for 12–18 months post-bariatric surgery?
A. Ineffective contraception
B. Increased sensitivity to oestrogen therapy (OCP or hormone replacement)
C. Increased risk of deep venous thrombosis
D. Foetal malnutrition secondary to maternal malnutrition
E. Increased risk of miscarriage

ANSWERS

Q1. Option C – Ileocaecal resection for Crohn's disease
Previous surgery may impact the technical feasibility of bariatric surgery. Previous gastric surgery (e.g., fundoplication) may prevent the placement of a gastric band or accurate gastric sleeve formation. Previous intestinal surgery or known small bowel adhesion disease may preclude any form of intestinal bypass. Intestinal diseases, such as Crohn's disease or extensive colitis, may render any form of bypass surgery intolerable and unwise. Those patients who have lost significant small intestinal length would also be unwise to consider intestinal bypass for weight loss. A diagnosis of hiatal hernia does not preclude bariatric surgery

Q2. Option C – Laparoscopic-assisted trans-gastric ERCP

There is an increased tendency for post-bariatric patients to develop gallstones due to altered bile acid kinetics and a change in diet. This is usually managed conservatively, but there is an indication here with the bile duct dilatation. In cases with acute cholangitis, CBD cannulation through interventional radiology may be an option, but this case can be managed by an expedited trans-gastric ERCP.

Q3. Option E – Roux-en-Y gastric bypass.

This patient has had a period of Tier 3 weight management and has a BMI of over 30. This in combination with a history of diabetes makes the patient a candidate for a Roux-en-Y bypass.

Q4. Option E – Emergency deflation of the band

Gastric bands are now very common, and we increasingly see more and more emergency presentations. This rare, but important complication leads to pain and intolerance of oral intake in the gastric band patient. It is due to a posterolateral prolapse of the fundus proximally 'up' through the band causing incarceration and if left untreated, proximal gastric strangulation. Diagnosis is by plain X-ray to identify the gastric band position and water-soluble contrast swallow. Immediate deflation, followed by prompt laparoscopic repositioning or removal of the band, is required.

Q5. Option D – Roux-en-Y gastric bypass

RYGB is now the predominant procedure worldwide (45% of procedures). The next most common procedures are sleeve gastrectomy (SG) (37.0%) and gastric band (10.0%).

Q6. Option B – A 42-year-old Persian female with a BMI of 31.7 kg/m^2 and new-onset diabetes

The NICE criteria on suitability for bariatric surgery for adults continue to be based on BMI criteria endorsed by the International Federation for the Surgery of Obesity and Metabolic Disorders (IFSO), National Institutes of Health and several other organisations:
- A BMI of >40 kg/m^2.
- A BMI of >35 kg/m^2 + significant comorbidity (e.g., type 2 diabetes mellitus (T2DM), hypertension, hyperlipidaemia, OSA, obesity hypoventilation syndrome, Pickwickian syndrome, non-alcoholic fatty liver disease (NAFLD), non-alcoholic steatohepatitis (NASH), pseudo-tumour cerebri, gastro-oesophageal reflux disease (GORD), asthma and functional disability).
- All appropriate non-surgical measures have been tried but have failed to achieve or maintain adequate, clinically beneficial weight loss for at least 6 months.
- The person has been receiving or will receive intensive management in a specialist obesity service.
- The person is generally fit for anaesthesia and surgery.
- The person commits to the need for long-term follow-up.
- As a first-line option (instead of lifestyle interventions or drug treatment) for adults with a BMI>50 kg/m^2 in whom surgical intervention is considered appropriate.

Option E – Twisting at the jejuno-jejunostomy
> Closing internal spaces at the time of RYGB reduces the incidence of internal hernia, but it is associated with a slightly higher incidence of re-operation due to kinking at the jejuno-jejunostomy anastomosis

Q7. Option E – Gastro-gastric fistula
> Approximately 3.0%–5.0% of RYGB patients develop marginal ulcers. Though the majority will present within 1–2 years, they can occur many years later. Typically, patients have persisting epigastric pain, with or without nausea and vomiting. Smoking, non-steroidal inflammatory drugs and *Helicobacter pylori* colonisation seem to be associated with an increased incidence of marginal ulcers. The diagnosis is by endoscopy. Treatment with a PPI with or without sucralfate, in conjunction with smoking cessation advice, usually results in prompt healing. It is important that patients undergo a check follow-up endoscopy to ensure healing as some ulcers do not heal on medical management. An underlying gastro-gastric fistula should be sought with a contrast X-ray swallow when an ulcer fails to heal.

Q8. Option E – Copper
> Neurological complications are rare after bariatric surgery and usually indicate a micronutrient deficiency. Vitamin B12, thiamine and copper constitute the most frequent deficiencies associated with neurological problems.

Q9. Option D – Roux-en-Y gastric bypass
> In a systematic review and meta-analysis of the effect of sleeve gastrectomy on GORD, the pooled incidence of new-onset GORD symptoms was 20.0%, with a strong suggestion of heterogeneity. The incidence of new-onset oesophagitis was about 6.3%. Most of these patients can be managed successfully with a PPI, but not lifelong, especially with metaplastic changes. Conversion to an RYGB usually improves symptoms in those with persistent symptoms despite PPI therapy.

Q10. Option B – Faster delivery to distal ileum post malabsorptive surgery stimulates enteroendocrine cells to release satiety hormones
> Gut peptides are secreted from EECs that reside within the intestinal epithelium and are often referred to as satiety hormones. Metabolic surgery can increase the number of gut peptide-expressing EECs (e.g., L cells) and, therefore, postprandial gut peptide secretion (e.g., GLP-1, GLP-2 and PYY). Patients with the highest postprandial levels of satiety hormones lose the most weight post-RYGB. Changes in nutrient concentrations (higher in the distal segments) and faster delivery to the distal ileum post-RYGB give stimulus to EECs to release these 'satiety' hormones, resulting in increased satiety, reduced food intake and sustained weight loss. In vertical sleeve gastrectomy (VSG), faster gastric emptying has been used to explain the rise in satiety hormones.
>
> Both PYY and GLP-1 act at the arcuate nucleus to suppress food intake but also via vagal afferents terminating at the nucleus tractus solitarius to signal satiety. GLP-1 also slows gastric emptying, inhibits glucagon release and acts on the pancreas to secrete insulin (incretin effect).

Q11. Option E – Rapid gastric emptying

Metabolic surgery has also been shown to result in obesity-related comorbidity improvement or resolution. The main mechanisms for this comorbidity resolution after bariatric surgery include

- Changes in eating behaviour and weight loss
- Gut hormones
- Bile acid kinetics
- Adipocyte-derived factors
- Anatomical factors.

Q12. Option D – A 16-year-old with a BMI of 38.9 kg/m^2

Bariatric surgery should only be considered in children/adolescents in bariatric centres that can offer specialist multidisciplinary paediatric bariatric services. The patients should have a BMI >40 kg/m^2 (or 99.5th percentile for respective age), have at least one comorbidity, have undergone a minimum of 6 months of supervised weight loss under a paediatric weight loss clinic, have skeletal and developmental maturity and have the ability to commit to medical and psychological assessment and commitment to postoperative multidisciplinary treatment.

Q13. Option A – A BMI of 51 kg/m^2

Pre-operative weight loss of at least 5% can reduce operative time and potentially operative risk, although this does not necessarily equate to a reduction in postoperative complications, except in patients with a BMI >55 kg/m^2, when it is believed to reduce postoperative mortality.

Q14. Option D – The American Society of Anaesthesiologists (ASA) physical status classification

To ascertain the level of risk and stratify patients' suitability for surgery, various risk assessment tools have been developed and validated. The most extensively validated tool is the ASA, which is used to ascertain anaesthetic risk. Several validated scores exist to assess surgical risk, including the OSMRS, the Edmonton Obesity Staging Score (EOSS) and King's Obesity Staging Score. The King's criteria use the mnemonic ABCDEFGHI and incorporate BMI and functional status into a scoring system. The EOSS has surpassed OSMRS as being a more comprehensive scoring system taking into account the severity of obesity-related comorbidity and is currently the preferred scoring system of BOMMS.

Q15. Option A – Fasting glucose of <6.1 mmol/L

Q16. Option A would not be considered to be diabetic. In T2DM patients, glycaemic control should be optimised preoperatively to a HbA1c of 6.5%–7.0% (47.5–53 mmol/mol; 7.8–8.6 mmol/L) and a fasting blood glucose level of 110 mg/dL (6.1 mmol/L). Patients may be considered for surgery at higher HbA1c levels of 7%–8% (53 mmol/mol–64 mmol/mL) if they have advanced microvascular or macrovascular complications, extensive comorbid conditions or long-standing poorly controlled diabetes despite all efforts.

Q17. Option D – Foetal malnutrition secondary to maternal malnutrition

All female patients should be advised against pregnancy for 12 months postoperatively due to the increased risk of foetal malnutrition secondary to maternal malnutrition and also be counselled regarding postoperative contraception. Additionally, oestrogen therapy (both contraception and hormone replacement therapy) should be discontinued before surgery to reduce deep vein thrombosis (DVT) risk.

2 Breast Surgery

*Hamed Noor Khan, Carol Norman,
and Rachel O'Connell*

Q1. In the diagnostic assessment of patients with known breast cancer, what is the most predictive parameter required?
   A. Tumour grade
   B. Tumour size
   C. Lymph node status
   D. ER and HER2 status
   E. All of the above

Q2. Routine MRI use should be considered in
   A. Patients with lobular neoplasia
   B. If breast density precludes accurate mammographic assessment
   C. Routine surveillance of post-operative patients
   D. In the preoperative assessment of patients with biopsy-proven invasive breast cancer or ductal carcinoma in situ (DCIS)
   E. All of the above

Q3. CT staging should be considered in
   A. Stage I breast cancer
   B. Stage II breast cancer
   C. Stage III breast cancer
   D. None of the above
   E. a, b, and c

Q4. In patients with bone symptoms and known breast cancer, which test is the most accurate in detecting bone metastasis?
   A. Tumour markers
   B. Plain film X-ray
   C. Isotope whole-body bone scan
   E. PET/CT
   F. None of the above

Q5. In a metastatic setting, in those who are hormone (ER+)-positive or HER2-negative and have not previously been on endocrine therapy, which regime could be considered first-line treatment
   A. Letrozole
   B. Letrozole with LHRH antagonists
   C. Letrozole in combination with CDK inhibitors
   D. Chemotherapy
   E. Anastrozole

DOI: 10.1201/9781003221234-2

Q6. Multifocal breast cancers
  A. Always need a mastectomy
  B. Are always in different quadrants
  C. Have a worse prognosis compared to unifocal cancers
  D. Accounts for 40% of all breast cancers
  E. None of the above

Q7. Periductal mastitis:
  A. is more common in smokers
  B. is polymicrobial with anaerobes and aerobes
  C. can be recurrent
  D. all of the above
  E. none of the above

Q8. Which statement is true?
  A. Ovarian suppression should be considered in young pre-menopausal ER-positive breast cancers requiring chemotherapy.
  B. Ovarian suppression should be considered in all pre-menopausal ER-positive breast cancers.
  C. Ovarian suppression should be considered in all young breast cancer cases requiring chemotherapy.
  D. Ovarian suppression is only indicated in a metastatic setting.
  E. None of the above

Q9. In nipple discharge, which statement is true?
  A. Can be divided into physiological and pathological
  B. Can be ignored if not bloody
  C. Can be ignored if initial investigations are negative
  D. Is a symptom of Paget's disease of the breast
  E. All of the above

Q10. In reduction mammaplasty, which pedicle results in retaining the most sensitivity to the nipple–areolar complex.
  A. Superior pedicle
  B. Superomedial pedicle
  C. Inferior pedicle
  D. Lateral pedicle
  E. Medial pedicle

Q11. A 49-year-old female presenting with radiological 2.3 cm, grade 3, ER–ve, HER2 +ve, and LN –ve,
  A. Should be considered for pre-surgical genetic testing
  B. Should be offered breast-conserving surgery
  C. Should be offered neoadjuvant chemotherapy and anti-HER2 therapy
  D. None of the above
  E. All of the above

Q12. In a breast surgical follow-up clinic, a patient with post-axillary node dissection presents with loss of sensation in the lateral aspect of the upper arm and reduction in the abduction of the shoulder joint, which structure has been injured?
A. Axillary nerve
B. Inter-costobrachial nerve
C. Thoraco-dorsal nerve
D. Nerve to serrates anterior
E. Median pectoral branch

Q13. In a breast surgical follow-up clinic, a patient with post-axillary node dissection presents with paraesthesia to the upper medial arm, which structure has been injured?
A. Axillary nerve
B. Intercosto-brachial nerve
C. Thoraco-dorsal nerve
D. Nerve to serrates anterior
E. Median pectoral branch

Q14. A 35-year-old lady has a 40 mm grade 3 invasive ductal carcinoma, triple negative, with two lymph nodes positive on ultrasound and core biopsy. Post-neoadjuvant chemotherapy, what is the recommended next step for the management of the axilla?
A. No axillary surgery
B. Axillary node clearance
C. Sentinel-Node Biopsy (dual technique)
D. Sentinel-Node Biopsy (single technique)
E. Sentinel-Node Biopsy and four-node sampling

Q15. A 50-year-old fit and well gentleman is diagnosed with a left breast, 20 mm grade 2 invasive ductal carcinoma hormone-positive, HER-2 negative, with normal lymph nodes on USS. What is the next step of management?
A. Primary endocrine therapy
B. Primary neoadjuvant chemotherapy
C. Wide local excision alone
D. Wide local excision with sentinel-node biopsy
E. Mastectomy and axillary surgery

Q16. A 50-year-old fit and well gentleman is diagnosed with a left breast, 20 mm, grade 2 invasive ductal carcinoma, hormone-positive, HER-2 positive, with normal lymph nodes on USS. What is the next step of management?
A. Primary endocrine therapy
B. Primary neoadjuvant chemotherapy
C. Wide local excision alone
D. Wide local excision with sentinel-node biopsy
E. Mastectomy and axillary surgery

Q17. A 50-year-old fit and well gentleman is diagnosed with a left breast, 49 mm, grade 2 invasive ductal carcinoma, which is hormone-negative and HER-2-negative, with normal lymph nodes on ultrasound. What is the most appropriate next step for management?
   A.   Neoadjuvant chemotherapy
   B.   Mastectomy and sentinel-node biopsy
   C.   Targeted therapy – Trastuzumab
   D.   Targeted therapy – Trastuzumab and Pertuzumab
   E.   Neoadjuvant chemotherapy and targeted therapy

Q18. A 52-year-old smoker presents for the third time to a clinic with a recurrent superficial wound with pustulent discharge, this area abuts the nipple–areolar complex. There is a green nipple discharge. In the management of this condition, which is the least likely modality of treatment?
   A.   Intravenous antibiotics
   B.   Regular wound dressing change
   C.   Stop smoking
   D.   Incision and drainage
   E.   Oral antibiotics

Q19. A 35-year-old lactating breastfeeding mother presents to the emergency department with right breast mastitis, which would be the most appropriate management?
   A.   Stop breastfeeding, ultrasound ± aspiration, IV antibiotics
   B.   Stop breastfeeding, ultrasound ± aspiration, PO antibiotics
   C.   Express milk and discard, ultrasound ± aspiration, PO antibiotics
   D.   Continue to breastfeed, ultrasound ± aspiration, PO antibiotics
   E.   Continue to breastfeed, ultrasound ± aspiration, IV antibiotics

Q20. Which of the following breast surgery procedures does not have a recommendation for the use of prophylactic antibiotics?
   A.   Therapeutic mammoplasty
   B.   Implant-based reconstruction
   C.   Standalone sentinel-node biopsy
   D.   Nipple surgery
   E.   Axillary node clearance

Q21. A 60-year-old lady has undergone a left-breast nipple-sparing mastectomy and implant-based reconstruction. She has had a protracted inpatient stay. You are the general surgery consultant on call over the weekend and have been informed by your registrar that the patient has a severe breast infection, is systemically unwell and the implant is visible through the wound. What is the most appropriate management?
   A.   IV antibiotics, wound washout on the ward, dressings
   B.   IV antibiotics, replacement of dressings, await breast surgery review post-weekend
   C.   IV antibiotics, washout ± debridement in theatre, exchange of the implant.
   D.   IV antibiotics, washout ± debridement in theatre, removal of the implant.
   E.   IV antibiotics, wound washout on the ward, placement of PICO or Vac dressing.

Q22. A 35-year-old patient, with no personal breast cancer history, has a family history of her mother who suffered from breast cancer at the age of 39. She has no other family history of breast or ovarian cancer. Which is the most appropriate management?
  A. Annual mammograms to start at 40
  B. No annual surveillance mammogram, reassure and discharge
  C. Annual surveillance mammogram, commence immediately
  D. MRI+annual mammograms
  E. Genetic testing

Q23. A patient undergoes genetic testing and has a 45%–85% lifetime risk of breast cancer and a 10%–30% risk of ovarian cancer. For which of the following predictive genes has she tested positive?
  A. CHEK 2
  B. PALB 2
  C. BRCA 1
  D. BRCA 2
  E. TP53

Q24. A patient has a 5 cm (benign) phyllodes tumour excised with >1 cm margin on all sides. What is the next step of management?
  A. Radiotherapy
  B. Annual clinical follow-up
  C. Chemotherapy
  D. Sentinel-node biopsy
  E. Discharge

Q25. Post-wide local excision and sentinel-node biopsy, a patient's histology results returns as T2 33 mm, N1 and M0. She has a grade 3 invasive ductal carcinoma which is ER8-, PR8- and HER-2 negative. What is her NPI score?
  A. 3.42
  B. 4.42
  C. 4.66
  D. 5.66
  E. 5.88

ANSWERS

Q1. Option D – ER and HER-2 Status.
  Although all of the criteria are required, the question asks about the most important one. The NICE (National Institute of Clinical Excellence) Guidelines on Early and locally advanced breast cancer advises oestrogen receptor (ER), progesterone receptor and human epidermal growth receptor 2 (HER-2) status for all invasive breast cancers simultaneously at the time of initial histopathological diagnosis.

Q2. Option B – If breast density precludes accurate mammographic assessment.
  The NICE guidelines suggest the use of magnetic resonance imaging (MRI) in patients with increased breast density. Lobular neoplasia is essentially a benign

condition and consists of atypical lobular hyperplasia and lobular carcinoma in situ. The NICE recommends that MRI should not be routinely used in invasive ductal carcinoma or DCIS or in the post-operative surveillance of breast cancer patients. If a patient is diagnosed with invasive lobular cancer and they wish to have breast conservation, then an MRI should be considered as lobular cancer is more likely to be multifocal. The NICE states 'Offer MRI of the breast to people with invasive breast cancer: if there is a discrepancy regarding the extent of disease from clinical examination, mammography and ultrasound assessment for planning treatment, if breast density precludes accurate mammographic assessment, to assess the tumour size if breast-conserving surgery is being considered for invasive lobular cancer'.

Q3. Option C – Stage III

From the literature, true metastases were detected in 1 (0.2%), 0 (0%) and 24 (6.0%) patients with stage I, II, and III disease, respectively. Chest CT, however, upstaged 6.0% of stage III patients to stage IV. Of note, there are no specific guidelines on staging in patients diagnosed with breast cancer from the NICE. Therefore, this question may be considered controversial as some clinicians will only stage if it appears that there are multiple abnormal lymph nodes rather than just one.

Q4. Option D – PET/CT

Although isotope bone scintigraphy is the usual test due to wide availability and reduced radiation exposure its method of detection is via increased blood flow in the osteoblastic activity of the metastatic bone disease. Its sensitivity is about 70%. CT PET is the most accurate with an accuracy of up to 90%. Its detection is through glycogen avid osteolytic actions of bone metastasis.

Q5. Option C – Letrozole in combination with CDK inhibitors

Palbociclib with an aromatase inhibitor for previously untreated, hormone receptor-positive, HER-2-negative, locally advanced or metastatic breast cancer is the treatment advised by the NICE Technology appraisal guidelines [TA495]

Q6. Option C – Have a worse prognosis compared to unifocal cancers

Breast-conserving surgery may be safely performed in the case of MF/MC cancer provided that the disease can be adequately excised with a good cosmetic result Breast cancers are defined as multifocal when there is more than one distinct tumour within the same quadrant of the breast (MF) and multicentric when multiple cancers develop in different quadrants of the breast (MC). Results of a recent study indicate that MF/MC cancers have a negative impact on prognosis and are related to higher loco-regional and distant relapse independently from the type of surgery performed. Most studies suggest an MF rate of 15%.

Q7. Option D – all of the above

Smoking, obesity and DM appear as risk factors for periductal mastitis. However, it is not conclusive that smoking is the cause of the condition. Bacterial contamination of the periductal system is noted with both anaerobes and aerobes.

Q8. Option A – Ovarian suppression should be considered in young pre-menopausal ER-positive breast cancers requiring chemotherapy.

This was the conclusion of the SOFT trial. Adding ovarian suppression to tamoxifen did not provide a significant benefit in the overall study population. However, for women who were at sufficient risk for recurrence to warrant adjuvant chemotherapy and who remained pre-menopausal, the addition of ovarian suppression improved disease outcomes. Further improvement was seen with the use of exemestane plus ovarian suppression.

Q9. Option A – Can be divided into physiological and pathological.

Although malignant nipple discharge is usually bloody, clear and serous discharge may also signify an underlying malignant cause. In post-menopausal women, an underlying malignant cause can still be found in 10% of cases whose initial investigations were negative. Although some women may describe discharge from Paget's, this is usually an ooze from the skin surface rather than a direct discharge from the nipple ducts. Nipple discharge has traditionally been broken down into physiological and pathological. The latter includes symptoms of spontaneity, bloody clear or serous colour and unilateral and uniductal.

Q10. Option D – Lateral pedicle

Lateral pedicle preserves both the deep and superficial branch of the fourth intercostal nerve, which is the main nerve to the nipple–areolar complex.

Q11. Option C – Should be offered neoadjuvant chemotherapy and anti-HER-2 therapy

Fast-track genetics should be considered for those under 60 and triple negative. For all other breast cancers, consider fast-track service in those deemed as young (<45 years of age).

Neoadjuvant chemotherapy (NACT) plus pertuzumab–trastuzumab is appropriate for patients with high-risk HER2-positive EBC (tumour diameter ≥ 2 cm, and/or node-positive disease). Patients with node-negative disease and tumour diameter <2 cm are candidates for upfront surgery followed by paclitaxel for 12 weeks plus 18 cycles of trastuzumab, with the option to add pertuzumab (if pN+). In the absence of high-risk genetic mutation (>10% BRCA1 and 2 carrier status), breast-conserving surgery should be offered to all patients if possible, but this will depend on patient and surgeon choice and preference

Q12. Option A – Axillary nerve

This is a very rare nerve injury as the brachial plexus and therefore axillary nerve should not be encountered during axillary node dissection. The main structure affected by injury to the axillary nerve is the deltoid muscle; therefore, there will be a loss of abduction of the shoulder joint. Sensory loss will be in the region of the lateral upper arm (deltoid).

Q13. Option B – Intercosto-brachial nerve

This is the typical distribution of sensory nerve loss with injury to the intercosto-brachial nerve. This is sometimes sacrificed during axillary dissection, particularly in heavily disease-burdened axillae.

Q14. Option E – Sentinel-node biopsy and four-node sampling

In this situation, two lymph nodes (N1 as part of the TNM (tumour-node-metastases) classification) are positive. The ABS (Association of Breast Surgeons) guidelines recommend that these patients can be safely considered for sentinel-node biopsy after neoadjuvant chemotherapy. Four nodes should be removed with dual mapping with patent blue dye and a labelled colloid radioisotope such as technetium-99m. There are alternatives to technetium-99m, but in the UK, this is the current standard.

Q15. Option E – Mastectomy and axillary surgery

The ASCO guidelines describe the following components of the management of breast cancers for men and women to be largely the same: (1) use of gene expression profile testing to guide adjuvant treatment decision-making (oncotype DX and prognostic tests), (2) primary surgery, (3) adjuvant chemotherapy, (4) adjuvant radiation therapy, and (5) chemotherapy for advanced/metastatic disease.

Q16. Option E – Mastectomy and axillary surgery

You have not been given the option of targeted biological therapy, e.g., trastuzumab, with neoadjuvant taxane-based chemotherapy (this would be the likely next step in management in MDT [Multidisciplinary Team]). Therefore, the next best is the answer required, a lateral thinking technique used in the exam.

Q17. Option A – Neoadjuvant chemotherapy

This patient has a triple negative T2 cancer and would be eligible for neoadjuvant chemotherapy *(NICE guidelines)*. He is HER-2-negative, so targeted therapy is not required. He would then proceed to mastectomy and sentinel-node biopsy using a dual technique with four nodes sampled.

Q18. Option D – Incision and drainage

This patient presents with periductal mastitis (PDM). This is a complex benign breast disease with a prolonged course and a high risk of recurrence after treatment. Conservative and medical management are the first line of management with the use of antibiotics and regular dressings. There is an increased risk in smokers and immunosuppressed patients including diabetics and lactating mothers. In those who persistently smoke, PDM is recurrent and there is poor and prolonged wound healing after surgical intervention. Patients should be strongly encouraged to stop smoking, which can often relieve symptoms.

There are many available interventional or surgical treatments, but none are widely accepted. This includes ultrasound-guided aspiration, breast duct irrigation, and minor and major excisions including plastic surgery techniques for large lesions with concerns about breast appearance. Incision and drainage and minor excision with primary closure alone should be avoided.

Q19. Option D – Continue to breastfeed, ultrasound±aspiration, PO antibiotics

NICE CKS guidelines advise that lactating women with mastitis or breast abscesses should continue to breastfeed if possible (including from the affected breast). If this is too painful, or the infant refuses to breastfeed from the affected breast, it is advised that the women express milk until she is able to resume breastfeeding from that breast.

It is not mentioned that the patient is systemically unwell, and this therefore negates the need for intravenous antibiotics.

Ultrasound is performed to rule out the presence of an abscess/deep collection which may require aspiration.

Q20. Option C – Standalone sentinel-node biopsy

Prophylactic antibiotics are beneficial to breast cancer patients undergoing surgery to prevent surgical-site infections. ABS summary guidelines suggest the following use of prophylactic antibiotics in a variety of breast and axillary operations:

Recommendation	Procedures
No prophylaxis	Standalone sentinel-node biopsy
	Excision of benign lump
Consider single-shot prophylaxis	Simple mastectomy
	Wide local excision
	Axillary node clearance
	Therapeutic mammoplasty
	Breast reduction/mastopexy
	Nipple surgery
	All repeat/revision surgery
Single dose at induction, second intraoperative dose if >4 hours of operating time, maximum three doses	All implant-based surgery.
	All autologous breast reconstruction procedures

Source: https://associationofbreastsurgery.org.uk/media/64256/final-antibiotic-prophylaxis.pdf

Q21. Option D – IV antibiotics, washout±debridement in theatre, removal of the implant.

You are the *general surgery consultant* on call. In the question, you are not given the most likely option to contact the breast surgery team for a take back to the theatre. Therefore, in a strategy that can be used to answer a number of FRCS questions, you would choose the safest option given. In this case, it would be to treat her sepsis and systemic symptoms and remove the source of infection by placing her onto CEPOD theatre for a general anaesthetic wound washout±debridement and removal of the implant.

Q22. Option A – Annual mammograms to start at 40

This patient falls into category B1 surveillance according to The Institute for Cancer Research and Royal Marsden Hospital NHS Foundation Trust protocols. She should have annual mammograms from 40 to 50 years and 3-yearly mammograms as part of the NHS breast screening programme from 50 to 70.

Other patients included in category B1 surveillance include patients with one male first-degree relative with breast cancer at any age, one female first-degree relative and one female second-degree relative with breast cancer at any age, and three female first-degree or second-degree relative with breast cancer at any age.

Category B2 surveillance patients require annual mammograms from 40 to 60 and 3-yearly mammograms from 60 to 70. There should be a discussion of chemoprevention – daily tamoxifen to reduce the risk of breast cancer.

Q23. Option D – BRCA2

The lifetime risk of breast cancer (to 80 years) in BRCA 1 patients is 60%–90% and an ovarian cancer lifetime risk of 40%–60%. For BRCA 2, this is 45%–85% and 10%–30%, respectively.

Faults in the PALB2 gene increase the risk of developing breast cancer by the age of 70 by 50%. CHEK 2 mutation corresponds to a twofold increase in the risk of breast cancer. Li Fraumeni syndrome, a fault in the TP53 gene, increases the risk of developing breast cancer, bone sarcoma, acute myeloid leukaemia, lymphoma, soft tissue sarcoma, brain tumours (glioblastomas) and adrenocortical carcinomas. Ninety percent of females develop breast cancer by age 60.

Q24. Option B – Annual clinical follow-up

Phyllodes tumours are rare fibro-epithelial lesions and make up less than 1% of all breast tumours. They can be benign, borderline or malignant. More than 50% (60%–75% in published evidence) are benign. This is a benign tumour that has been completely excised with clear margins; no adjuvant therapy is required and the patient should be followed up clinically as there is an increased risk of recurrence (overall 21%). Local recurrences generally develop within 2–3 years.

Borderline and malignant tumours are treated as sarcomas and should be referred to the regional sarcoma unit. The use of radiotherapy, chemotherapy and sentinel-node biopsy is decided on an individual patient basis.

Q25. Option D – 5.66

The Nottingham Prognostic Index (NPI) calculates the prognosis of patients following breast cancer surgery.

To calculate, NPI = tumour size in cm $\times 0.2$ + histological grade [1–3] + number of positive lymph nodes [1 = 0 nodes; 2 = 1–3 nodes; 3 >3 nodes].

3.3 cm $\times 0.2 = 0.66$, $0.66 + 3$ (grade) $= 3.66$, $3.66 + 2$ (N1 disease) $= 5.66$

A good prognosis is < 3.4, a moderate prognosis is 3.41–5.4 and a poor prognosis is >5.4.

NPI is not commonly used in practice but is a frequent exam question.

FURTHER READING

http://www.icr.ac.uk/
https://www.cancerresearchuk.org/about-cancer/causes-of-cancer/inherited-cancer-genes-and-increased-cancer-risk/inherited-genes-and-cancer-types
https://www.ncbi.nlm.nih.gov/books/NBK539895/

Hassett M.J.; Somerfield M.R.; Baker E.R.; Cardoso F.; Kansal K.J.; Kwait D.C.; Plichta J.K.; Ricker C.; Roshal A.; Ruddy K.J.; Safer J.D.; Van Poznak C.; Yung R.L; Giordano S.H. Management of Male Breast Cancer: ASCO Guideline. *Journal of Clinical Oncology*, Volume 38, Issue 16. https://ascopubs.org/doi/full/10.1200/JCO.19.03120. Epub 2020 Feb 14. PMID: 32058842.

Limaiem F.; Kayshap S. (2022). Phyllodes Tumor. In: *StatPearls* [Internet]. Treasure Island, FL: StatPearls Publishing. https://www.ncbi.nlm.nih.gov/books/NBK541138/

NICE Clinical Knowledge Summaries. (2021). Mastitis and breast abscess. Mastitis and abscess. Available from https://cks.nice.org.uk/mastitis-and-breast-abscess

Xu H.; Lv Y.; Mu W.; Yang Q.; Fu H.; Li Y.; Liu R.; Fan Z. (2021). Treatments for Periductal Mastitis: Systematic Review and Meta-Analysis. *Breast Care*, Volume 17, pp. 55–62.

3 Colorectal Surgery

Arnab Bhowmick, Aya Musbahi,
Muhammad Rafay Sameem Siddiqui,
Stephen Holtham, and John Corson

Q1. A 47-year-old patient attends your clinic after a colonoscopy was performed for a family history of bowel cancer. She has a family history of bowel cancer with her father being diagnosed with rectal cancer at 51 years. Her latest colonoscopy was normal. What would you advise in terms of follow-up?
A. Screening only
B. Colonoscopy every 5 years
C. Flexible sigmoidoscopy annually with interval colonoscopies at 5 years
D. One further colonoscopy at 5 years and if a negative discharge
E. CEA 6 monthly

Q2. A 46-year-old man attends your clinic after a colonoscopy performed 12 months earlier for a family history of bowel cancer. He has a family history of bowel cancer with his father being diagnosed at 63, a paternal aunt diagnosed at 61 and a half-brother from his father's side being diagnosed at 57. His latest colonoscopy was normal. What would you advise in terms of follow-up?
A. Screening only
B. Colonoscopy after 5 years
C. Colonoscopy after 4 years
D. Colonoscopy after 3 years
E. Annual colonoscopy

Q3. A 47-year-old attends your clinic with a change in bowel habits and is sent for a colonoscopy. She is found to have 12 polyps in the colon varying in size between 5 and 10 mm with histology confirming low-grade dysplastic adenomas. After a discussion with a colleague, you decide to send her for germline testing which comes back negative. How would you approach her endoscopic surveillance?
A. Colonoscopy in 24 months
B. Colonoscopy in 12 months with dye spray
C. Colonoscopy in 12 months without dye spray
D. Screening only
E. None – consider subtotal colectomy

Q4. A neighbour comes to your house for dinner one evening. He tells you that he was adopted when he was a young boy and now that he is 25 is looking for his biological family. During the conversation, he tells you that he has recently discovered that his biological father was diagnosed with bowel cancer at 40, his paternal uncle at 53, and his grandad at 60. He has recently had a genetic test which has identified that he is a PMS2 carrier. He knows you are a colorectal surgeon and asks what he should do.

 DOI: 10.1201/9781003221234-3

A. Colonoscopy and OGD biannually from age 25
B. Colonoscopy from age 25 and OGD from age 50 every 2 years
C. Colonoscopy biannually from age 25
D. Colonoscopy biennially from age 25
E. None of the above

Q5. A worried mother comes to your clinic having been referred to you by her GP. She has a 9-year-old son who has been bullied by discolouration of his lips and dark blue spots over his nose. He had a colonoscopy which showed multiple polyps which the surgeon she spoke to described as having a lot of fibrous tissue and lots of blood vessels in it. She is worried about his brother who is 4 years old. On examination of her youngest child, you do not identify any abnormality except some blue spots around his mouth. What would you advise?
A. Colonoscopy when the youngest child turns 15
B. Video capsule endoscopy only when the child turns 8
C. OGD only when the child turns 8
D. Video capsule endoscopy and OGD when the child turns 8
E. Colonoscopy and OGD when the child turns 15

Q6. A 40-year-old lady has an EUA and biopsy for an anal lesion which is excised and sent to pathology. Histology confirms AIN 3 diagnosis. What are the next steps?
A. Discussion at anal cancer MDT and review by a specialist pathologist
B. Referral for high-resolution anoscopy and acetic acid-targeted biopsies
C. HIV testing
D. Commencement of imiquimod
E. Cryoablation

Q7. A lady with AIN 3 is referred for regular surveillance. What interval of surveillance is likely to be recommended by the MDT?
A. 6-monthly intervals for 2 years
B. 12-monthly intervals for 5 years
C. 6-monthly intervals for 5 years
D. 3-monthly intervals for 3 years
E. 12-monthly intervals for 10 years

Q8. A lady with AIN diagnosed 6 months earlier comes back with a 1 cm lesion which is biopsied. Cancer is confirmed, and staging confirms T1 N0 M0. MDT recommends excision by the anal canal surgeon. Excision is performed with no compromise to sphincters with a 1 mm margin. What are the next steps?
A. Continued surveillance follow-up
B. Adjuvant CRT
C. Re-excision of margins
D. Recruitment to the ACT3 arm of the PLATO trial
E. Discharge

Q9. Which of the following statements is true with regard to the detection of colorectal carcinomas in patients whose symptoms were suggestive?
 A. Colonoscopy has a higher sensitivity to CT colonography and double-contrast barium enema
 B. Colonoscopy has equal sensitivity to CT colonography but higher than double-contrast barium enema
 C. All three investigations have the same sensitivity
 D. CT colonography has a higher sensitivity than colonoscopy
 E. Double-contrast barium enema is a superior investigation to CT colonography

Q10. A 55-year-old patient is invited for one off-flexible sigmoidoscopy for screening. What reduction in CRC-related mortality does this screening tool represent?
 A. 11%
 B. 21%
 C. 31%
 D. 41%
 E. 51%

Q11. A 56-year-old patient with COPD is admitted as an emergency with obstructing mid-sigmoid cancer and a CT scan that shows bilobar indeterminate liver lesions. What would be the optimum management option?
 A. Open Hartmann's and biopsy of the liver lesions
 B. Defunctioning colostomy and biopsy of the liver lesion
 C. Defunctioning ileostomy and MRI of the liver
 D. Laparoscopic sigmoid colectomy
 E. Colonic stent and further workup of the patient as a bridge to elective resection

Q12. Which of the following is NOT associated with increased 30-day mortality in elective colorectal cancer surgery in the elderly?
 A. Male gender
 B. Use of laparoscopy
 C. Advancing age
 D. Charlson comorbidity index >3
 E. Emergency surgery

Q13. Which type of pouch is associated with less nighttime defecation and less use of antidiarrhoeals?
 A. W pouch
 B. J pouch
 C. S pouch
 D. U pouch
 E. M pouch

Q14. Which of the following statements about pouch-anal anastomoses is true?
 A. Stapled-pouch anal anastomosis is inferior to hand-sewn in terms of pouch function
 B. Stapled and hand-sewn have similar pouch function outcomes

    C.   Stapled-pouch anal anastomosis is superior to the hand-sewn one in terms of pouch function

    D.   Cuffitis is an issue with hand-sewn anastomoses

    E.   Pouch dysplasia cannot be reduced with a mucosectomy

Q15. Which of the following statements regarding pouch surgery is true?
    A.   A diverting ileostomy is necessary in all cases
    B.   A diverting ileostomy can be omitted in selected cases
    C.   A diverting ileostomy has no impact in reducing pelvic sepsis
    D.   There is no difference in the leak rate between diverting ileostomy and no diverting ileostomy after pouch surgery
    E.   Diverting ileostomies are not associated with increased morbidity compared to no ileostomies

Q16. Which of the following is the most common late complication of pouch surgery?
    A.   Small bowel obstruction
    B.   Pouch fistula
    C.   DVT
    D.   Strictures
    E.   Pouch cancer

Q17. A 30-year-old patient 3 years after the formation of a pouch presents with urgency, bloody diarrhoea and abdominal pain. Endoscopic investigations and histology confirm pouchitis. She has no allergies. What should be the first-line antibiotic in this instance?
    A.   Amoxicillin
    B.   Ciprofloxacin
    C.   Metronidazole
    D.   VSL 3
    E.   Erythromycin

Q18. The risk of cancer in the rectum after ileorectal anastomosis (IRA) for IBD at 20 years is:
    A.   5%
    B.   7%
    C.   9%
    D.   14%
    E.   30%

Q19. Which of the following is an absolute contraindication to a continent (Kock pouch) ileostomy?
    A.   Obesity
    B.   Small bowel Crohn's disease
    C.   Marginal small bowel length
    D.   Intra-abdominal desmoids
    E.   Failed pouch surgery

Q20. A 36-year-old lady with Crohn's presents with a non-healing fistula in the 3 o'clock position. What would be the optimum management in this case?
  A. Multimodal surgical treatment with setons and medical therapy with infliximab
  B. Seton management initially with medical therapy reserved for failure
  C. Fistula plug
  D. LIFT procedure
  E. Fistulotomy

Q21. An otherwise fit and well patient with duodenal Crohn's disease presents with gastric outlet obstruction secondary to a duodenal stricture. Which of the following represents first-line management?
  A. Endoscopic balloon dilatation
  B. Strictureplasty
  C. Whipple's procedure
  D. Gastrojejunostomy
  E. Duodenal stent

Q22. Which of the following is not associated with lower recurrence rates after ileocolic resection for Crohn's disease?
  A. Kono S anastomosis
  B. Five ASAs
  C. Long disease duration
  D. Mesenteric excision
  E. Smoking

Q23. A 76-year-old gentleman with UC is being managed in the medical ward and has nine stools per day. His CRP is 100, and he is being managed with steroids. What is his risk of needing a colectomy on this index admission?
  A. 25%
  B. 50%
  C. 60%
  D. 70%
  E. 85%

Q24. A 76-year-old gentleman with UC is being managed in the medical ward and has nine stools per day. His CRP is 100 and he is being managed with steroids. The patient refuses an operation and would like to try rescue medical therapy. He has a history of previous tuberculosis. Which medication would be a relative contraindication in this setting?
  A. Ciclosporin
  B. Infliximab
  C. Vedolizumab
  D. Adalimumab
  E. Istekizumab

Q25. Which of the following is not an evidence-based management option for d-IBS?
   A. Increased fibre intake
   B. Tricyclic antidepressants
   C. Low FODMAP diet
   D. Loperamide
   E. Cognitive behavioural therapy

Q26. A 45-year-old lady is referred with slow transit constipation confirmed on an X-ray transit study. A defecating proctogram has excluded prolapse or rectal intussusception. She has tried dietary fibre and various laxatives and has good compliance. What management option can be considered next?
   A. Prucalopride
   B. Linaclotide
   C. Biofeedback
   D. ACE
   E. Subtotal colectomy

Q27. Which of the following is the most common type of caecal volvulus?
   A. Bascule
   B. Lateral rotation
   C. Axial ileocolic volvulus
   D. Saggital volvulus
   E. Internal herniation

Q28. A fit and healthy 60-year-old lady presents with CT showing caecal volvulus. What represents the best management option?
   A. Right hemicolectomy
   B. Caecopexy
   C. Caecostomy
   D. Colonoscopic detorsion
   E. Neostigmine

Q29. Which of the following stomas are associated with the highest risk of parastomal hernia formation?
   A. Loop colostomy
   B. Loop ileostomy
   C. End colostomy
   D. End ileostomy
   E. Caecostomy

Q30. An ITU patient is being treated for acute colonic pseudo-obstruction with neostigmine. Which of the following does not represent a contraindication to its use?
   A. Advanced age
   B. Recent MI
   C. Second-degree heart block
   D. Chronic kidney disease
   E. Arrhythmias

Q31. A 25-year-old female is referred to you from gastroenterology with terminal ileal Crohn's disease. Current medical therapy is with azathioprine. Small bowel MR scanning has shown 10 cm of the strictured thickened terminal ileum with high signal inflammatory change and mild pre-stenotic dilatation. Symptoms are continuous right iliac fossa pain and diarrhoea. The patient smokes 20 cigarettes per day and has no other comorbidity. Her abdomen is unremarkable on examination. The most appropriate surgical opinion would be:

A.   Counsel and consent for surgical resection – standard right hemicolectomy with terminal ileal resection

B.   Discuss ileo-caecectomy as an option, but explore the possibility with MDT of biological therapy with infliximab, as well as smoking cessation

C.   Start high-dose prednisolone based on MR scan and symptoms, and schedule surgery when the dose is down to 5 mg/day with post-operative metronidazole for 3 months

D.   Organise colonoscopy and terminal ileal balloon dilatation

E.   No discussion necessary about surgery as no obstruction symptoms or fistulation – discharge back to gastroenterology

Q32. In the small bowel, Crohn's fibrostenotic strictures may be treated with strictureplasty. In which of the following situations should a strictureplasty not be performed?

A.   A 4 cm stricture with 75% fat encroachment 15 cm from Duodeno-jejunal flexure

B.   A 4 cm stricture 10 cm from the ileo-caecal junction with active bowel wall inflammation present

C.   A 3 cm stricture at distal ileum with associated phlegmon and interloop abscess

D.   A 4 cm stricture at mid-ileum – patient on regular infliximab infusions

E.   A 4 cm recurrent stricture in a patient with multiple strictures

Q33. In restorative proctocolectomy, a one-stage procedure with defunctioning loop ileostomy could be appropriately performed for a patient in which of the following circumstances?

A.   Familial adenomatous polyposis with fully penetrant phenotype and no rectal sparing

B.   Severe ulcerative colitis maintained in remission with vedolizumab and oral steroids

C.   Acute severe colitis with high-dose steroid therapy but where the albumin level is still in the normal range

D.   Crohn's colitis in remission with rectal sparing

E.   Indeterminate colitis with perianal fistulae – setons already inserted and all sepsis controlled

Q34. A 56-year-old patient who underwent urgent subtotal colectomy and ileostomy for acute severe colitis 3 months ago attends your clinic for review. There is a discharging sinus on the peri-stomal skin around 5 mm from the mucocutaneous junction. The discharge is similar to ileal effluent. Stoma bags are not adhering satisfactorily, and the peristomal skin looks erythematous with patchy desquamation. What would be the most appropriate next step?

    A.   Urgent incision and drainage of discharging area with hydrogen peroxide

    B.   CT scan of the abdomen followed by fluoroscopic fistulogram

    C.   Small bowel MR with full oral bowel preparation

    D.   Urgent elective Ileoscopy under anaesthetic proceeding to the mobilisation of stoma/resection

    E.   Admit for urgent exploratory Laparotomy

Q35. A 45-year-old male with known Crohn's proctitis presents with a 3 cm perianal abscess. He is currently managed with oral olsalazine. At operation, there is a fluctuant abscess which you incise and drain. On sigmoidoscopy/proctoscopy, a low intersphincteric fistula becomes apparent, encompassing the lower fifth of the internal sphincter. There is also severe proctitis. The appropriate next action would be to:

    A.   Lay open the fistula give post-operative antibiotics and repeat EUA for 3 months

    B.   Insert a loose seton, pack the cavity and arrange an in-patient pelvic MR

    C.   Insert a cutting seton, pack the cavity and re-examine with EUA in 48 hours

    D.   Insert a loose seton, pack the cavity and get a gastroenterology opinion

    E.   Apply negative pressure dressing and start steroid enemas

ANSWERS

Q1. Option A – Screening only.

    The BSG and ACPGBI updated their guidelines in late 2019 and divide family history risk into average, moderate and high. This is a more simplified classification than the previous guidelines. For those with average risk with no family history or those that do not fulfil the moderate or high-risk criteria, the surveillance should follow that of the national screening protocol. The current national screening guidelines in the UK are to have 2 yearly FIT tests from 56 years to 74 years. Note that the age has expanded to 56 years in 2021. Prior to 2021, the start age was 60. People who are at moderate risk of developing colorectal cancer should have a colonoscopy at 55 years. Moderate-risk cancers include people with one first-degree relative under 50 with colorectal cancer or two first-degree relatives (in a first-degree kinship) with colorectal cancer at any age; at least one of these should be a first-degree relative of the person seeking advice on surveillance. High-risk individuals include those with at least three affected relatives (within a first-degree kinship) diagnosed with colorectal cancer at any age, and at least one is a first-degree relative of the person seeking advice. These patients should have a colonoscopy every 5 years until 75 years.

Q2. Option C – Colonoscopy after 4 years.

    This patient is considered to be a high-risk candidate with three affected individuals in a first-degree kinship. He had a colonoscopy 12 months earlier, and the protocol would be every 5 years after the age of 40. He therefore needs another colonoscopy in 4 years to adhere to the protocols advised in the guidelines. Of note, if the family history criteria fit the Lynch criteria, then surveillance may be offered according to Lynch-like syndrome or Lynch syndrome (if the MMR variant is confirmed).

Q3. Option B – Colonoscopy in 12 months with dye spray.

This clinical scenario represents a typical picture of patients with multiple colorectal adenomas (MCRAs) The guidelines would suggest that those with more than ten adenomas and MUTYH/APC negative should have a colonoscopy in 12 months. At the subsequent colonoscopy, if no polyps are seen which are more than 10 mm, surveillance can be increased to biennial colonoscopies. Additionally, the use of dye spray helps categorise these polyps according to their phenotype.

Q4. Option E – None of the above.

This patient would fulfil the criteria of Lynch syndrome. He has had genetic testing and was found to be a PMS2 carrier. His risk is therefore slightly lower than if he was an MLH1 or MSH2 gene carrier. The recommended age of surveillance is 2 yearly colonoscopies after the age of 35. If he had an MLH1 or MSH2 mutation, then the surveillance would commence at the age of 25. The original surveillance was 2 yearly OGDs from the age of 50, but these have been changed in the recent guidelines and are now only offered within the context of a clinical trial.

Q5. Option D – Video capsule endoscopy and OGD when the child turns 8.

The child in question is a relative of someone with likely Peutz–Jegher syndrome. Hamartomas on histology are typically described as cystic dilation of mucus-filled glands, prominent bands of fibrous stroma, and a rich vascular network. The surveillance for these patients would include OGD, capsule endoscopy and a colonoscopy from age 8. Peutz–Jegher syndrome is associated with an STK11 gene variant. Small bowel surveillance should continue every 3 years. If the baseline colonoscopy and OGD are normal, then further scopes can recommence at the age of 18; however, if polyps are present, then a 3-yearly surveillance protocol should be adopted. These are the protocols for asymptomatic patients; however, in symptomatic patients, investigations should commence earlier.

Q6. Option A – Discussion at anal cancer MDT and review by a specialist pathologist.

The ACPGBI guidelines mandate that all new diagnoses of ANI 2 and 3 (HSIL) be discussed at a specialist anal cancer MDT. Female patients with AIN should be screened for VIN, CIN and VAIN. In addition, recurrent or multifocal AIN should prompt HIV testing. The use of anoscopy in clinical practice routinely has not been validated outside of clinical trials. Topical therapies such as imiquimod and cryoablation have been used with varying results in the regression and treatment of HSIL.

Q7. Option C – 6 monthly intervals for 5 years.

Surveillance is aimed at detecting and performing a biopsy of any new lesions with the aim of early detection. There is significant heterogeneity amongst multiple guidelines with regard to the frequency and nature of AIN surveillance.

Q8. Option D – The ACT3 trial is designed as a non-randomised, phase II multi-centre trial in patients with T1N0 anal margin cancers and is part of a much larger study (PLATO).

Patients with T1N0 cancers are treated with wide local excision. Those with margins of greater than 1mm are referred for surveillance. Those with 1 mm or smaller margins undergo chemoradiotherapy according to a predefined treatment strategy (41.4Gy in 23 fractions with concurrent day 1 MMC and capecitabine 825 mg/mg bd on days of radiotherapy). There is a paucity of evidence with regard to what is the optimum margins and whether close margins necessitate adjuvant therapy.

Q9. Option B – Colonoscopy has equal sensitivity to CT colonography but higher than that of double-contrast barium enema.

This question refers to the SIGGAR trial, the UK Special Interest Group in Gastrointestinal and Abdominal Radiology. This trial randomised patients with symptoms suggestive of colorectal cancer to CT colon versus double-contrast barium enema, with the end point being the detection of cancer of polyps greater than 1 cm. The other group were randomised to colonoscopy or CT colon with an end point being the necessity of further investigation after one or other. The main findings were that CT colons detected more cancers and larger polyps than double-contrast barium enemas and that the detection rate between CT colons and colonoscopy showed no significant difference (11.4% vs 10.7%) but that CT colons generated more investigations than colonoscopy. The authors and a previous meta-analysis concluded no significant difference in the sensitivity of both tests, leading the ACPGBI to recommend either investigation for symptoms suggestive of colorectal cancer.

Q10. Option C – 31%.

The bowel scope programme is based on a large RCT by Atkin and colleagues in 2010 who randomised just over 170,000 patients to receive flexible sigmoidoscopy between the ages of 55 and 64 or no intervention. The study found that the incidence of colorectal cancer was less by 23% in the intervention group and mortality related to CRC less by 31% compared to the control group.

Q11. Option E – Colonic stent and further workup of the patient as a bridge to elective resection.

Recent studies have shown the advantages to self-expanding metal stents as a bridge to surgery in malignant left-sided bowel obstructions such as reduced stoma rates and morbidity rates as well as increased chance of having a laparoscopic operation; however, stent complications remain a problem. A study by Mora-Lopez et al, 2020, demonstrated no difference in oncological outcomes between those bridged via SEMS and those who did not and had surgery. The CREST trial is one of the largest RCTs comparing SEMS as a bridge to surgery and emergency surgery. A total of 246 patients were randomised between 2009 and 2014. Thirty-day post-operative mortality (5.3% vs 4.4%) and the length of hospital stay [15.5 days (IQR 10–26) vs 16 days (10–27)] were similar with stenting and surgery. Stenting achieved relief of obstruction in 82% of patients and reduced stoma formation and 69% emergency surgery vs 45% with stenting as a bridge to surgery (p<0.001). There was no significant difference in the mortality in 3-month and 12-month quality-of-life parameters.

Q12. Option B – Use of laparoscopy.

A study by Faiz and colleagues in 2011 reported outcomes in the elderly having colorectal resections. This showed the 30-day mortality of those above 85 years old to be double their younger counterparts. It also showed male gender and more comorbidities indicated by the Charlson comorbidity index to be independent risk factors. The use of laparoscopy was associated with lower 30-day mortality.

Q13. Option A – W pouch.

Although the J pouch is the most commonly used modern pouch, three randomised trials have compared J and W pouches. All pouch types in a meta-analysis had similar complication rates. The J pouch is favoured due to greater technical ease in formation. Although few long-term studies, there remain concerns over the massive distention of a W pouch.

Q14. Option C – Stapled-pouch anal anastomosis is superior to the hand-sewn one in terms of pouch function.

A large meta-analysis of both techniques demonstrated superior post-operative pouch function outcomes. It is also technically easier.

Q15. Option B – A diverting ileostomy can be omitted in selected cases.

Diversion ileostomy has been shown to reduce the incidence of pelvic sepsis which is a risk factor for pouch dysfunction. A diversion ileostomy can also reduce the incidence of a pouch leak. However, a diverting ileostomy is in itself associated with morbidity, admissions with small bowel obstruction and dehydration. The ACPGBI guidelines recommend that diverting ileostomies can be omitted in a select few patients with fewer risk factors who have been optimised with any signs and symptoms of pelvic sepsis and pouch picked up early.

Q16. Option A – Small bowel obstruction.

Small bowel obstruction occurs in 25% of patients after pouch surgery, usually adhesional in nature. Incomplete evacuation and straining may be indicative of a stricture. This may be at the level of the anastomosis or proximal to it which should raise the question of Crohn's disease. DVT is surprisingly common in this cohort with 6% of patients developing symptomatic venous thrombosis and many developing portal vein thrombosis.

Q17. Option C – Metronidazole.

Most patients should be treated within 7–10 days. The refractory and relapsing disease may require long-term antibiotics. VSL 3 has been shown in a randomised controlled trial to maintain remission. This may be due to alterations in bacterial flora after pouch formation.

Q18. Option D – 14%.

Careful counselling and selection as well as surveillance of patients for IRA should be performed. Females wishing to preserve their fertility represent a group who may wish to opt for this surgery rather than IPAA which can reduce fertility by up to 50%, probably due to pelvic adhesions. Dysplasia is associated with ulcerative colitis and increases over time, leading to cancer in the retained rectum. Patients should be counselled regarding the need for continued surveillance of the rectum and the risks associated with rectal preservation. Those with previous dysplasia in colonic specimens should be counselled against IRA. The risk of cancer is 2% at 10 years. No clear surveillance guidelines exist, but it is recommended that biopsies and annual flexible sigmoidoscopy are undertaken 8–10 years post-op with any finding of dysplasia an indication to do a proctectomy. Counselling and consent are vital in this situation.

Q19. Option B – Small bowel Crohn's disease.

The other options represent relative contraindications for Kock pouch ileostomy. There has been interest in this procedure in individuals who have either failed pouch surgery or who have contraindications to pouch surgery such as poor sphincters and continence. This procedure is not commonly performed in the UK but is common in Scandinavian countries despite even widespread use of IPAA. Around 50 cm of the small bowel is required to form the continent ileostomy. Desmoids in cases of FAP are relative contraindications due to their ability to increase in size with the trauma of surgical intervention. Obesity can also preclude the formation of the ileostomy due to intra-abdominal thickness, especially in cases of short small bowel mesentery.

Q20. Option A – Multimodal surgical treatment with setons and medical therapy with infliximab.

Surgery for Crohn's perianal fistulas should prioritise sphincter and continence preservation. A systematic review showed greater healing rates for multimodal surgical therapy with setons and medical therapy (55%) than surgical treatment alone (25%). There is a paucity of evidence with regard to fistula plugs, fibrin glue or the ligation of intersphincteric track (LIFT) procedure. Advancement flaps are associated with high failure rates and incontinence. Video-assisted anal fistula treatment shows initial promise in treatment but long-term outcomes are awaited.

Q21. Option A – Endoscopic balloon dilatation.

Strictures in D1/D2 related to Crohn's disease can be treated in the first instance endoscopically with balloon dilatation. Reported success rates are up to 80% with a 2% perforation rate. For refractory and relapsing cases, gastrojejunostomy or strictureplasty can be considered. There is little evidence to support one technique over the other. There is little evidence to support vagotomy. PPI and *Helicobacter pylori* eradication should be considered in all cases. Duodenal Crohn's fistulas requiring repair may necessitate duodenal repair and a Thal patch repair with jejunal serosa may be preferable to an omental patch repair in such cases.

Q22. Option E – Smoking.

Smoking is associated with higher recurrence rates as well as short disease duration. 5-ASA use is associated with lower recurrence rates. Patients should be referred for smoking cessation in cases of recurrent disease in smokers. There has been much interest in the Kono S anastomosis. This is a hand-sewn functional end-to-end antimesenteric anastomosis which has been shown in small studies to reduce the recurrence of Crohn's after bowel resection. Larger studies and long-term outcomes are awaited. Radical mesenteric excision to reduce recurrence in a contentious area but not currently advocated.

Q23. Option E – 85%.

   This question relates to the Travis criteria that states that on day 3, 85% of patients with more than eight stools on that day, or a stool frequency between three and eight together with a CRP >45 mg/L, would require colectomy.

Q24. Option B – Infliximab.

   Infliximab risks reactivating latent TB. A careful history should be taken and a chest X-ray and testing where there is doubt. Cyclosporin should not be used in hypertensives.

Q25. Option A – Increased fibre intake.

   Increased fibre intake is not indicated and can make symptoms worse in diarrhoeal-predominant IBS. There is good evidence for TCAs such as amitriptyline but is unlicensed. Guidelines recommend low FODMAP diets as well as loperamide. There is also good evidence for CBT and some evidence for hypnotherapy. Cutting down on caffeine and sorbitol should also be encouraged.

Q26. Option A – Prucalopride.

   Prucalopride is a 5HT4 agonist which has shown promising results in functional constipation resistant to other laxatives. It acts to increase peristalsis and reduce transit time. Linaclotide is recommended for use in those with IBS components to their constipation as per the Rome IV criteria. Biofeedback is recommended in cases with pelvic floor dysfunction characterised by a group of conditions such as anismus, paradoxical contraction of the puborectalis muscle or spastic pelvic floor syndrome. Good success rates are reported, but limited success is achieved in those with slow transit constipation. Surgery should only be reserved in highly selected cases who have failed to progress with conservative measures and in whom neuro-gastroenterological disorders have been excluded.

Q27. Option C – Axial ileocolic volvulus.

   The most common type of caecal volvulus is axial ileocolic volvulus (90%) with bascule volvulus forming the other 10%. In axial ileocolic volvulus, the caecum rotates up and to the left upper quadrant with a characteristic empty right iliac fossa. In the bascule, the caecum flips up and anteriorly with an absence of axial rotation. Bascule type is less likely associated with strangulation than axial ileocolic volvulus.

Q28. Option A – Right hemicolectomy.

   Surgical resection is usually mandated due to the high risk of gangrene and ischaemic in the stretched caecum. It is advisable intra-operatively not to detort the caecum so as not to release toxins into the circulation. Caecopexy is associated with high recurrence rates. Detorsion is associated with 75% recurrence rates but caecostomy can be considered in very frail and high-risk patients as a temporary measure as it has an associated recurrence rate of 20%.

Q29. Option C – End colostomy. Controversy exists as to the prevention of parastomal hernias. There remains a belief that herniation is reduced when stoma formation is through the rectus rather than lateral to it but studies remain conflicted and inconclusive in this regard. Prophylactic mesh is thought to be preventative.

Q30. Option A – Advanced age.

Contraindications to neostigmine use include a known allergy to the medication, recent myocardial infarction, reactive airway disease, chronic kidney disease and uncontrolled arrhythmias. A serious side effect is a symptomatic bradycardia which may need atropine and thus needs to be given in monitored settings.

Q31. Option B – Discuss ileo-caecectomy as an option, but explore the possibility with MDT of biological therapy with infliximab, as well as smoking cessation.

It would be reasonable to offer surgery, but in view of the stricture having a distinct inflammatory component still, there may still be mileage in further medical therapy with a biological agent

Q32. Option C – 3 cm stricture at distal ileum with associated phlegmon and interloop abscess.

Bowel wall phlegmon and localised sepsis would contraindicate strictureplasty

Q33. Option A – Familial adenomatous polyposis with fully penetrant phenotype and no rectal sparing.

FAP patients require a full proctocolectomy due to cancer risk, and a three-stage procedure (subtotal colectomy, then proctectomy and pouch with covering ileostomy, followed by ileostomy closure) would not be appropriate due to the risk of interval cancer in the rectum

Q34. Option D – Urgent elective ileoscopy under anaesthetic proceeding to the mobilisation of stoma/resection.

It is most likely that there is fistulating Crohn's disease in the ileum comprising the stoma. Ileoscopy will identify the disease. The stoma can then be mobilised and resected. Given the skin deterioration, it is appropriate to act quickly rather than embark on investigations.

Q35. Option D – Insert a loose seton, pack the cavity and get a gastroenterology opinion.

This option allows the best drainage combined with a minimal risk to sphincters as well as addressing the proctitis which needs better control.

FURTHER READING

Alam NN, White DA, Narang SK, Daniels IR, Smart NJ. Systematic review of guidelines for the assessment and management of high-grade anal intraepithelial neoplasia (AIN II/III). *Colorectal Disease* 2016 Feb;18(2):135–146.

Atkin W, Dadswell E, Wooldrage K, Kralj-Hans I, von Wagner C, Edwards R, Yao G, Kay C, Burling D, Faiz O, Teare J. Computed tomographic colonography versus colonoscopy for investigation of patients with symptoms suggestive of colorectal cancer (SIGGAR): A multicenter randomised trial. *The Lancet* 2013 Apr 6;381(9873):1194–1202.

Brown SR, Fearnhead NS, Faiz OD, Abercrombie JF, Acheson AG, Arnott RG, Clark SK, Clifford S, Davies RJ, Davies MM, Douie WJ. The Association of Coloproctology of Great Britain and Ireland consensus guidelines in surgery for inflammatory bowel disease. *Colorectal Disease* 2018 Dec;20:3–117.

Cubiella J, Carballo F, Portillo I, et al. Incidence of advanced neoplasia during surveillance in high- and intermediate-risk groups of the European colorectal cancer screening guidelines. *Endoscopy* 2016;48:995–1002.

Dalal RL, Shen B, Schwartz DA. Management of pouchitis and other common complications of the pouch. *Inflammatory Bowel Diseases* 2018 Apr 23;24(5):989–996.

Derikx LA, de Jong ME, Hoentjen F. Short article: Recommendations on rectal surveillance for colorectal cancer after subtotal colectomy in patients with inflammatory bowel disease. *European Journal of Gastroenterology & Hepatology* 2018 Aug 1;30(8):843–846.

Faiz O, Haji A, Bottle A, Clark SK, Darzi AW, Aylin P. Elective colonic surgery for cancer in the elderly: An investigation into postoperative mortality in English NHS hospitals between 1996 and 2007. *Colorectal Disease* 2011 Jul;13(7):779–785.

Hill J, Kay C, Morton D, Magill L, Handley K, Gray RG, CREST Trial Collaborative Group. CREST: Randomised phase III study of stenting as a bridge to surgery in obstructing colorectal cancer—Results of the UK ColoRectal Endoscopic Stenting Trial (CREST). *Journal of Clinical Oncology* 34(15):3507.

Langman G, Loughrey M, Shepherd N, Quirke P. Association of Coloproctology of Great Britain & Ireland (ACPGBI): Guidelines for the Management of Cancer of the Colon, Rectum and Anus (2017)-Pathology Standards and Datasets. *Colorectal Disease* 2017 Jul;19:74–81.

Lightner AL. Duodenal Crohn's disease. *Inflammatory Bowel Diseases* 2018 Feb 16;24(3):546–551.

Liu JJ, Venkatesh V, Gao J, Adler E, Brenner DM. Efficacy and safety of neostigmine and decompressive colonoscopy for acute colonic pseudo-obstruction: A single-center analysis. *Gastroenterology Research* 2021 Jun 19;14(3): 157–164.

Lopez N, Ramamoorthy S, Sandborn WJ. Recent advances in the management of perianal fistulizing Crohn's disease: Lessons for the clinic. *Expert Review of Gastroenterology & Hepatology* 2019 Jun 3;13(6):563–577.

Lovegrove RE, Constantinides VA, Heriot AG, Athanasiou T, Darzi A, Remzi FH, Nicholls RJ, Fazio VW, Tekkis PP. A comparison of hand-sewn versus stapled ileal pouch anal anastomosis (IPAA) following proctocolectomy: A meta-analysis of 4183 patients. *Annals of Surgery*. 2006 Jul;244(1):18.

Monahan KJ, Bradshaw N, Dolwani S, Hereditary CRC Guidelines eDelphi Consensus Group, et al. Guidelines for the management of hereditary colorectal cancer from the British Society of Gastroenterology (BSG)/Association of Coloproctology of Great Britain and Ireland (ACPGBI)/United Kingdom Cancer Genetics Group (UKCGG). *Gut* 2020;69:411–444. https://www.bsg.org.uk/wp-content/uploads/2019/12/Guidelines-for-the-management-of-hereditary-colorectal-cancer.full_.pdf

Mora-López L, Hidalgo M, Falcó J, Serra-Pla S, Pallisera-Lloveras A, Garcia-Nalda A, Criado E, Navarro-Soto S, Serra-Aracil X. Long-term outcomes of colonic stent as a "bridge to surgery" for left-sided malignant large-bowel obstruction. *Surgical Oncology* 2020 Dec 1;35:399–405.

Myrelid P, Block M, editors. *The Kock Pouch*. Springer International Publishing; 2019.

Okeny PK. Caecal volvulus. In: Garbuzenko D. (Ed.), *Intestinal Obstructions*. London: IntechOpen; 2020. https://www.intechopen.com/chapters/71272 doi:10.5772/intechopen.91311

Renehan AG, Muirhead R, Berkman L, McParland L, Sebag-Montefiore D. Early stage anal margin cancer: Towards evidence-based management. *Colorectal Disease* 2019;21:387–391.

Renkonen-Sinisalo L, Sipponen P, Aarnio M, et al. No support for endoscopic surveillance for gastric cancer in hereditary non-polyposis colorectal cancer. *Scandinavian Journal of Gastroenterology* 2002;37:574–577.

Sherman J, Greenstein AJ, Greenstein AJ. Ileal J pouch complications and surgical solutions: A review. *Inflammatory Bowel Diseases* 2014 Sep 1;20(9):1678–1685.

Smalley W, Falck-Ytter C, Carrasco Labra A. AGA clinical practice guidelines on the laboratory evaluation of functional diarrhoea and diarrhoea-predominant irritable bowel syndrome in adults (IBS-D). *Gastroenterology* 2019 Sep;157(3):851–854.

Sobrado CW, Corrêa IJ, Pinto RA, Sobrado LF, Nahas SC, Cecconello I. Diagnosis and treatment of constipation: A clinical update based on the Rome IV criteria. *Journal of Coloproctology (Rio de Janeiro)* 2018 Apr;38:137–144.

Styliński R, Alzubedi A, Rudzki S. Parastomal hernia–current knowledge and treatment. *Videosurgery and Other Miniinvasive Techniques* 2018 Mar;13(1):1.

Travis S, Satsangi J, Lémann M. Predicting the need for colectomy in severe ulcerative colitis: A critical appraisal of clinical parameters and currently available biomarkers. *Gut* 2011 Jan 1;60(1):3–9.

Yamamoto T. Factors affecting recurrence after surgery for Crohn's disease. *World Journal of Gastroenterology: WJG* 2005 Jul 14;11(26):3971.

4 Critical Care and Emergency Surgery

*Michael Courtney, Mitesh Sharma,
Arnab Bhowmick, Christophe Thomas,
Hazim Eltyeb, Ioannis Gerogiannis,
and Mohamed Baguneid*

Q1. A 70-year-old male presents with right iliac fossa pain. Examination reveals RIF rebound tenderness, with a temperature of 37.8°C, a pulse of 102 bpm, a BP of 130/80, and blood tests show a WCC of 13 and a CRP of 55. A CT abdominal scan reveals an inflamed appendix with a very small volume of free fluid and a thickened caecal pole. The patient has a background of severe heart failure within a walking distance of 20 m. He is also anticoagulated with warfarin for atrial fibrillation. The most appropriate treatment should be
  A. Reverse anticoagulation with vitamin K and operate – laparoscopic appendicectomy and inspection of caecal pole at operation
  B. Analgesia and referral to a palliative care pathway given the patient's advanced comorbidity
  C. Broad-spectrum intravenous antibiotic therapy only, discussing a significant risk of recurrence even if treatment successful
  D. Reverse anticoagulation with prothrombin concentrate followed by urgent open appendicectomy and palpation of caecal pole
  E. Urgent CT colonogram to assess right colon before any further decision

Q2. A 48-year-old male is diagnosed with sigmoid diverticulitis. A CT scan shows a 3.5 cm pericolic abscess with small gas locules extending out 4 cm from the bowel wall. The patient is pyrexial at 39°C, with a pulse of 96 bpm and a BP of 130/70 and has localised severe tenderness on palpation in the left lower quadrant. Inflammatory markers show a CRP of 96. The best option for management would be:
  A. Percutaneous drainage of abscess, nil by mouth and parenteral nutrition
  B. Intravenous co-amoxiclav and exploratory laparotomy within 24 hours if no improvement
  C. Oral ciprofloxacin and metronidazole for 2 weeks
  D. Immediate laparoscopy for source control with peritoneal lavage
  E. Intravenous co-amoxiclav with monitoring of clinical signs

Q3. Regarding the use of self-expanding metallic stents in malignant large bowel obstruction:
  A. Mortality is reduced by at least 10% compared to urgent surgery
  B. Stents are strictly contraindicated where anti-angiogenic chemotherapy may be required

DOI: 10.1201/9781003221234-4

   C.   Successful relief of obstruction is expected in around 70% of cases

   D.   Uncomplicated stenting appears to be as oncologically safe at 3–5 years as emergency surgery

   E.   Stents can only now be recommended in palliative cases

Q4. A 72-year-old male presents with mild-to-moderate fresh rectal bleeding to the emergency department. According to the Oakland score, factors important in predicting re-admission risk are:

   A.   Passing clots, cardiac disease, aspirin therapy

   B.   Confirmed diverticular disease, passing clots, <3 hours between bleeds

   C.   >3 days history, no piles on proctoscopy

   D.   Mixture of dark and fresh blood, >2 comorbidities

   E.   age > 70, blood pressure, digital rectal exam findings

Q5. A 35-year-old female presents with a 48-hour history of right upper-quadrant pain. She is otherwise systemically well on admission but has a pyrexia of 37.9°C with positive Murphy's sign on palpation. Liver function tests show a deranged liver function with ALP 190, GGT 165, ALT 88 (all IU/L), and bilirubin 6 mmol/L. Ultrasound scan shows a thickened oedematous gall bladder with multiple calculi. The CBD diameter is 3.5 mm. What is the most appropriate plan?

   A.   Laparoscopic cholecystectomy with on-table cholangiogram

   B.   Manage conservatively, then out-patient MRCP – if CBD is clear, proceed to cholecystectomy

   C.   Urgent endoscopic ultrasound followed by delayed laparoscopic cholecystectomy if LFTs settle

   D.   Open cholecystectomy with bile duct exploration

   E.   Urgent ERCP with sphincterotomy/balloon trawl of CBD followed by laparoscopic cholecystectomy

Q6. Which of the following is not a true statement regarding maintenance of patient normothermia during abdominal surgery, when compared with hypothermia

   A.   Wound infection rate is reduced by two-thirds

   B.   Cardiovascular complications are reduced threefold

   C.   The anion gap is cut by 40%

   D.   Reduces risks of intraoperative bleeding

   E.   Reduces the length of stay

Q7. Which of the following is true for arterial line monitoring of blood pressure during surgery

   A.   The waveform is characterised by the tricrotic notch

   B.   A 'swinging' arterial trace may indicate hypovolaemia

   C.   Pulse pressure is more accurate with a sphygmomanometer

   D.   A 500 mL bag of saline is attached to the line at 150 mmHg pressure

   E.   Area under the arterial waveform curve is continuously calculated to give mean arterial pressure

Q8. A 56-year-old male is to undergo laparotomy for small bowel obstruction via a midline incision. An epidural infusion is placed before induction of general anaesthesia. Which of the following statements best describes epidural analgesia for abdominal surgery?
  A. An epidural can be inserted safely in bacteraemia if antibiotics are to be given on induction
  B. The infusion is placed deep into the ligamentum flavum
  C. Epidural haematoma occurs in around 8% of patients and is mostly asymptomatic
  D. Hypotension may occur due to the inhibition of acetylcholine
  E. Opioid infusion via the epidural is contraindicated

Q9. An 80-year-old female with dementia undergoes in-patient orthopaedic surgical treatment for a lower limb fracture. Three days into the admission her abdomen has painlessly distended and tense. Digital rectal examination reveals a dilated gas-filled rectum. A subsequent CT abdominal scan shows no mechanical obstruction but the caecum is 13 cm in diameter. Her right iliac fossa is markedly tender with localised peritonism, and the abdomen is tense and tympanitic. She is pyrexial at 38.2°C, her pulse rate is 96 bpm and her blood pressure is 110/70. The blood picture shows a WCC of 22 and the CRP is 110. Assuming that the patient is fit enough for operative or endoscopic treatment, what is the most likely treatment required?
  A. Immediate endoscopic decompression
  B. Caecostomy under general anaesthetic
  C. Laparotomy, subtotal colectomy and ileostomy
  D. Laparoscopic transverse colostomy
  E. Laparotomy ileo-caecectomy and ileostomy

Q10. You attend the trauma resuscitation of a multiply injured 23-year-old motorcyclist found at the side of the road. The patient has a GCS of 13 and maintains his airway. The respiratory rate is raised at 28, and there is shallow breathing on both sides on chest auscultation with severe chest wall tenderness on the right side. The abdomen is tender and contused centrally and in the epigastrium. A pelvic binder is in situ. Both lower limbs are contused but with no external haemorrhage. The blood pressure on arrival is 96/50 with a pulse of 124 bpm. One unit of packed cells is rapidly transfused. The blood pressure thereupon rises to 105/70. Your suggestion for appropriate next steps will be:
  A. Abdominal and thoracic FAST scans. If negative, then immediate CT head
  B. Bilateral thoracotomies, chest drains and then abdominal FAST scan
  C. Transfer to a CT scanner for chest, abdomen and pelvis CT
  D. Transfer to the operating theatre for urgent laparotomy
  E. Chest X-ray and urgent echocardiography to exclude pericardial haemorrhage

Q11. You are asked to prescribe maintenance IV fluids to a 35-year-old female post-operative patient after open cholecystectomy. The patient is euvolaemic with normal serum electrolytes and has a BMI of 27. She has not resumed oral fluid/food intake yet. The most appropriate prescription would be:
  A. 55–65 mL/kg/day of water and 2 mmol/kg/day of potassium, sodium and chloride and 25 g/day of glucose

B. 125 mL/h Ringer's lactate then re-check electrolytes after 24 hours
C. 100 mL/h 0.9% saline with 20 mmol potassium in every other litre bag
D. 25–30 mL/kg/day water, 1 mmol/kg/day potassium, sodium and chloride, and 50–100 g/day glucose
E. Ringer's lactate alternating with 0.9% saline at 125 mL/h until oral fluids were tolerated

Q12. A 65-year-old man with a BMI of 39 kg/m^2 is admitted to the emergency surgical team with acute abdominal pain and nausea. He says that this pain appeared 6 months ago with less intensity, occurring once per month. However, as he says, yesterday became more intense and it is unbearable. He has a history of Roux-en-Y gastric bypass (RYGB) done 2 years ago. His preoperative BMI was 53 kg/m^2; WBC: 10.3, CRP: 5 and Lac: 1.3. What is the most appropriate next step for the management of this patient?
A. CT scan of the abdomen and pelvis
B. Diagnostic laparoscopy
C. Gastroscopy
D. Analgesia and PPIs
E. Ultrasound scan of the abdomen

Q13. A 53-year-old woman presents with a past medical history of type 2 diabetes mellitus, with a BMI of 33 kg/m^2 and multiple episodes of perianal abscesses drained previously. She presents with fever and perianal discomfort, haemodynamically stable with a heart rate of 97, a blood pressure of 100/65 mmHg, a WBC of 22 and a CRP of 400. On clinical examination, the perianal area is very tender and erythematous, but there is no sign of an obvious abscess. What is the most appropriate first step for the management of this patient?
A. Antibiotics and conservative management
B. Incision and drainage
C. CT scan of the pelvis
D. MRI of the pelvis
E. Aspiration with a needle

Q14. A 23-year-old male presented to A&E after an injury whilst playing rugby at a semi-professional level. The mechanism of injury was a direct hit to the central abdomen when the patient fell on the knee of one of his teammates after a collision. On presentation, his abdomen is soft, but there is generalised tenderness. The FAST scan showed a moderate amount of free fluid in Morrison's pouch and pelvis. WBC: 19 and CRP: 5. As the patient is haemodynamically stable, the A&E consultant asked for a CT of the abdomen and pelvis which showed a small amount of fluid in the right and left paracolic gutter and in the pelvis. No other pathology was found. What is the most appropriate next step for the management of this patient?
A. Antibiotics and repeat blood tests after 24 hours
B. Observe and repeat CT after 24 hours
C. Observe and repeat the FAST scan later that day
D. Diagnostic laparotomy
E. Diagnostic laparoscopy

Q15. The gastroenterology registrar is calling you for an 88-year-old woman who is under the medical team as she was admitted a few hours ago with continuous PR bleeding. She is on clopidogrel, and she is known to the oncology team with rectal cancer on radiotherapy. She is unstable with BP: 90/45 mmHg, HR: 117/minute, and on PR examination, she has a lot of fresh PR bleeding. The gastro team performed a rigid scope bedside and saw diffuse bleeding from the lower rectum and anal verge possibly secondary to radiation. Her last Hgb is 69, and there is a plan in place to transfuse her with vitamin K and TXA. What is the first course of action from the surgical point of view?

A. Just observe and transfuse
B. Arrange an urgent CT angiogram
C. Flexible sigmoidoscopy
D. EUA±proceed
E. Pack the rectum with gauze

Q16. A 65-year-old man with a history of AF on clopidogrel had an unwitnessed fall in his bathroom. He presented in A&E with abdominal discomfort and weakness. Asking him about the mechanism of the injury, he insists that the fall was minor, and he had hit only his upper abdomen on a small chair without any major pain or bruise. His vitals are T: 37, BP: 98/45 mmHg, and HR: 89 bpm and his blood tests revealed a Hgb of 70. He is haemodynamically stable, but on examination, the abdomen is rigid and tender. What is the most appropriate next step for the management of this patient?

A. Emergency laparotomy
B. Contact the haematologist for recombinant factor VII and emergency laparotomy
C. Transfuse and observe
D. CT scan of the abdomen and pelvis
E. Aggressive resuscitation with crystalloids

Q17. A 63-year-old man with T2DM presents with a 7-day history of erythema around an abdominal injection site. This has spread despite oral antibiotics. On examination, he is febrile, tachycardic and hypotensive, and there is 10 cm×15 cm of erythema beyond a previous marking line. The area is exquisitely tender, and there is a small area of necrosis at the injection site. What is the most appropriate treatment option?

A. Change to broad-spectrum oral antibiotic and discharge
B. Change to intravenous antibiotic and admit for observation
C. Change to intravenous antibiotic and CT with IV contrast
D. Change to intravenous antibiotic and arrange urgent debridement
E. Change to intravenous antibiotic and perform bedside incision of the necrotic skin

Q18. A 45-year-old male with a BMI of 45 presents at 22:00 hours with tender, irreducible abdominal swelling and vomiting. There is mild overlying erythema. CT with portal-venous contrast reveals a paraumbilical hernia containing fluid and a loop of jejunum, which is inflamed but enhanced. There is proximal small bowel obstruction. There is a case ongoing in the emergency theatre which is likely to finish in 1–2 hours. What is the most appropriate management?

    A.   NG tube and observation

    B.   NG tube and administration of gastrograffin

    C.   Attempted reduction of the hernia with IV analgesia and sedation

    D.   Admission for surgery during the night

    E.   Admission for surgery first in the morning

Q19. A 60-year-old man, with a history of hypertension and osteoarthritis, presents with perforation and is taken for a laparoscopic repair of a perforated anterior duodenal ulcer. What is the most likely aetiology of his ulcer?

    A.   Non-steroidal anti-inflammatory medication

    B.   Alcohol excess

    C.   *Helicobacter pylori* infection

    D.   Calcium-channel blocker side effect

    E.   Duodenal malignancy

Q20. A 65-year-old man with a background of ischaemic heart disease and a previous TIA presents with severe abdominal central abdominal pain of a 4-hour duration. On examination, he is distressed with significant pain, but his abdomen is soft with mild tenderness in all four quadrants. Blood tests reveal Hb 131, WCC 25, CRP 50, Amy 41, and lactate 7. What is the most appropriate next step?

    A.   IV fluid resuscitation, admit and repeat lactate

    B.   CT with portal-venous contrast

    C.   CT with arterial contrast

    D.   Diagnostic laparoscopy

    E.   Diagnostic laparotomy

Q21. A 70-year-old man presents to the hospital with abdominal pain 12 hours after a routine colonoscopy performed at another hospital. He tells you that a small polyp was removed, but otherwise, the test was normal. On examination, his abdomen is soft but tender, especially in the right lower quadrant. Blood tests show slightly raised inflammatory markers and normal haemoglobin. Plain chest and abdominal X-rays are unremarkable. What is the most appropriate management?

    A.   Reassurance and discharge

    B.   Admission for observation

    C.   CT abdomen with contrast

    D.   Diagnostic laparoscopy

    E.   Double-contrast enema

Q22. A 26-year-old man in police custody comes to the hospital 4 days after sustaining a penetrating rectal sustained whilst falling on a fence post. CT scan shows free extraperitoneal gas and fluid in the pelvis. He is taken for examination under anaesthesia, and there is a rectal defect approximately 1 cm in diameter. What is the most appropriate management?

    A.   Primary closure

    B.   Washout only

    C.   Endoscopic vacuum therapy

    D.   Diversion colostomy

    E.   Anterior resection

Q23. A 26-year-old female presents with a tender swelling to the breast, with surrounding erythema. She is a smoker but otherwise healthy. On examination, there is mild cellulitis to the breast with a firm central swelling. What is the most appropriate step?
   A. Analgesia and reassurance
   B. Analgesia and oral antibiotic
   C. Intravenous antibiotic and admission for observation
   D. Ultrasound-guided aspiration±culture
   E. Incision and drainage

Q24. A 40-year-old male presents to the A&E with a 2-week history of lower abdominal pain which has become worse over the last 2 days. On examination, he is tender in the right iliac fossa with a palpable fullness; the remainder of his abdomen is normal. Blood tests show Hb: 109, WCC: 19, and CRP: 98. What is your next step?
   A. Urgent laparoscopy
   B. Urgent CT with contrast
   C. Urgent ultrasound scan
   D. Urgent colonoscopy
   E. 2 ww colorectal referral

Q25. A 78-year-old female who is normally fit and healthy is admitted with a large rectal bleed. When you review her on the morning ward round, she has just had a further large bleed. Her current observations are HR: 110, BP: 100/70, and T: 36.5. What is the most appropriate investigation?
   A. In-patient sigmoidoscopy
   B. In-patient colonoscopy
   C. Out-patient colonoscopy
   D. CT with portal-venous contrast
   E. CT with arterial contrast

Q26. A 26-year-old female with Crohn's disease presents with perianal pain and discharge. On examination, there is a tender swelling at the 2 o'clock position and pus seeping from a punctum. What is the most appropriate management?
   A. EUA and incision and drainage
   B. EUA and seton
   C. IV antibiotics and observation
   D. IV antibiotics and MRI of the pelvis
   E. Urgent sigmoidoscopy

Q27. An 85-year-old female with ischaemic heart disease, atrial fibrillation and T2DM presents with peritonitis. A CT shows free intraperitoneal gas. She is taken to the theatre for a laparotomy, and there is four-quadrant turbid peritonitis due to a diverticular perforation. She requires inotropic support intra-operatively. What is the most appropriate next step?
   A. Washout and drainage
   B. Hartmann's procedure
   C. Sigmoid colectomy, primary anastomosis and ileostomy
   D. Sigmoid colectomy, primary anastomosis and no ileostomy
   E. Palliation

Q28. A 56-year-old female with a previous history of fibromyalgia presents at midnight with abdominal pain and bloating. A CT scan suggests likely caecal volvulus. What is the most appropriate treatment?
A. NG drainage
B. Oral contrast (e.g., gastrograffin)
C. Endoscopic detorsion
D. Caecopexy
E. Right hemicolectomy

Q29. A 26-year-old man, recently diagnosed with ulcerative colitis, is admitted to the hospital with acute severe colitis (as per Truelove and Witts criteria). What percentage of patients with acute severe ulcerative colitis require surgical intervention on their first admission?
A. 1%
B. 5%
C. 10%–20%
D. 25%
E. 50%

Q30. A 35-year-old man presents to the hospital with a 24-hour history of severe vomiting. He has now developed severe chest and upper abdominal pain. Blood tests including amylase are unremarkable and apart from a heart rate of 100/m, all clinical observations are normal. The chest X-ray is suspicious of surgical emphysema, although there is no obvious pneumothorax. What is the most likely diagnosis?
A. Pancreatitis
B. Gastritis
C. Mallory–Weiss syndrome
D. Boerhaave's syndrome
E. Gastric perforation

Q31. During routine elective laparoscopic cholecystectomy, significant brisk bleeding from the liver bed occurs which cannot be controlled by pressure or diathermy. What is the most appropriate next step?
A. On-table embolisation of hepatic artery
B. Packing of the liver with a haemostatic agent
C. Open conversion and liver packing
D. Laparoscopic pringle manoeuvre
E. Subtotal cholecystectomy and wedge resection of the liver

Q32. A 50-year-old man known to drink excessively is admitted with abdominal pain, bloating and vomiting. He reports being progressively less able to tolerate solids and now is dependent on liquid intake only. He was discharged 6 weeks ago following an attack of acute severe pancreatitis which was managed conservatively. He denies drinking alcohol post-discharge. On examination, there is a mass in the upper abdomen. Blood tests including amylase and CXR are normal. What is the most likely diagnosis?
A. Gastritis
B. Pancreatitis

    C. Pancreatic insufficiency
    D. Pancreatic pseudocyst
    E. Posterior DU perf

Q33. A 50-year-old female is admitted with abdominal pain 2 days after an elective laparoscopic cholecystectomy. CT shows fluid in the right upper quadrant. Diagnostic laparoscopy is performed, and it reveals bile in the subhepatic region; the cystic duct is visible, and a LIGACLIP was found appropriately placed. What is the next most appropriate step?
    A. Washout plus subhepatic wide-bore drain
    B. Intrahepatic cholangiogram + T-tube drainage via the cystic duct
    C. On-table ERCP
    D. Wedge liver resection
    E. Washout + post-op MRCP

Q34. A 45-year-old male is brought to the A&E following a road traffic collision; he is currently haemodynamically stable but complains of abdominal pain. A trauma CT reveals free fluid in the RUQ, but there is no clear solid organ injury. The patient is taken for a diagnostic laparoscopy which reveals bile in the RUQ and a gall-bladder perforation. What would the most appropriate management be?
    A. Conversion to laparotomy
    B. Laparoscopic cholecystectomy
    C. Laparoscopic cholecystectomy + intraoperative cholangiogram
    D. Laparoscopic cholecystectomy + intraoperative ERCP
    E. Laparoscopic cholecystectomy + PTC

Q35. A 50-year-old man (70 kg) is brought in via ambulance following a fall through a window, resulting in a large laceration to his arm. There is currently a tourniquet controlling the bleeding. His current observations are HR: 135, BP: 110/90, T: 35.8, and RR: 35. The GCS is 15. Approximately how much blood is he likely to have lost?
    A. 15% circulating volume
    B. 15%–30% circulating volume
    C. 30%–40% circulating volume
    D. 40%–50% circulating volume
    E. >50% circulating volume

Q36. A 45-year-old female with known liver cirrhosis and varices presents with haematemesis. She is currently stable, and her Hb is normal. What is the most appropriate next step?
    A. Urgent out-patient OGD
    B. IV PPI and admission for observation
    C. IV beta-blocker and admission for observation
    D. In-patient OGD with banding of varices
    E. Angiography and embolisation

Q37. A 75-year-old female, with a history of hypertension, attends the hospital with severe upper abdominal pain and repeated retching with vomitus containing only saliva. An urgent CT scan reveals a hiatus hernia and comments that the stomach is rotated with the greater curve lying superior to the lesser curve. She has been kept nil by mouth and IV fluid therapy is running. What is the most appropriate next step in management?

A. OGD
B. Wide-bore NG tube insertion bedside
C. Diagnostic laparoscopy + repair of hiatus hernia ± hiatal mesh
D. OGD + endoscopic gastropexy
E. Laparotomy + repair of hiatus hernia

Q38. An 18-year-old female presents following a fall from a horse. CT scan reveals a short (4 cm) capsular tear of the liver approximately 2 cm deep. She is stable and there are no other injuries. What is the most appropriate management option?

A. Admission for observation
B. Diagnostic laparoscopy
C. Laparotomy and packing
D. Angiographic embolisation
E. Open segmental resection

Q39. A 28-year-old female who is known to be an intravenous drug user presents with a swollen tender right gluteal region with crepitus and blisters. She had a pulse of 110 bpm, a BP of 110/60, a respiratory rate of 18/min and an O_2 saturation of 94% and was drowsy. What would be an appropriate management plan?

A. Give intravenous fluid bolus and broad-spectrum antibiotics. Arrange an urgent ultrasound scan to drain any collection
B. Give intravenous fluid bolus and broad-spectrum antibiotics. Take the patient to the theatre to debride the right gluteal wound once the patient has been fasting for 6 hours
C. Commence sepsis 6 bundles as the patient has sepsis based on the qSOFA score and take the patient to theatre immediately
D. Give intravenous fluid bolus, high-flow oxygen and broad-spectrum antibiotics. Check lactate and take the patient urgently to the theatre for debridement
E. Patient needs to be transferred to the intensive care unit immediately for fluids and intravenous broad-spectrum antibiotics until her infection resolves

Q40. A 78-year-old man is 3 days following an elective sigmoid colectomy for a malignant polyp. He has had no urine output from his urinary catheter for 12 hours and experiencing pain in his lower abdomen. His pulse is 98 bpm, BP is 160/90, temperature is 37.1°C, RR is 16/min and O_2 saturation is 96% on air. Which statement is most likely to be correct:

A. He is likely to have a pre-renal acute renal injury from hypovolaemia and needs a fluid bolus and reassess his urine output in 2 hours
B. His abdominal pain indicates that he has an anastomotic leak and developing sepsis with renal failure
C. He is likely to be in urinary retention and should have his urinary catheter flushed or changed
D. He needs to have an urgent CT scan with contrast to assess for an anastomotic leak or ureteric injury
E. He may have sustained the bilateral ureteric injury during his surgery and should have an urgent laparotomy

Q41. A 48-year-old female patient who was admitted with a diabetic foot infection underwent debridement of her forefoot and angioplasty of her posterior tibial and peroneal arteries 2 days ago. She was found to be oliguric for the past 24 hours and her blood tests just returned with Na: 138 mmol/L, K+: 6.9 mmol/L, Urea: 25 mmol/L, and creatinine: 385 mmol/L. An ECG demonstrated widened QRS complexes. What is the best course of action?

A.   Repeat her urea and electrolytes and consider transfer to the high-dependency unit

B.   Give 10 mL of 10% calcium gluconate, start salbutamol nebuliser and 500 mL of 10% Dextrose with 10 units of fast-acting insulin. Transfer to a high-dependency unit and plan for renal replacement therapy (RRT)

C.   Start salbutamol nebulisers and give oral calcium resonium. If there is no improvement, then she will need urgent RRT (haemofiltration or haemodialysis)

D.   Patient should go immediately for RRT

E.   Check patients' blood gases; if the patient has metabolic acidosis, then give sodium bicarbonate and Calcium Resonium.

Q42. A 28-year-old man was involved in a high-speed RTA as an unrestrained front-seat passenger arrives at the emergency department. His airway was clear. He was brought on a spinal board with neck restraints. He had a large wide-bore cannula in both antecubital fossae. His respiratory rate was 24/minute with an oxygen saturation of 94% on high-flow oxygen through a standard venturi mask. His pulse was 110 bpm and in sinus rhythm with a BP of 110/60. His GCS was 14/15. Chest X-ray confirmed fractures to the left first, second and third ribs associated with a large left-sided pneumothorax and a widened mediastinum. What would be an appropriate management plan:

A.   Perform rapid intubation and then place bilateral chest drains and transfer to the intensive care unit for cardiac monitoring

B.   Place a left-sided chest drain in the left fourth intercostal space and arrange an urgent CT trauma of the chest, abdomen and pelvis

C.   Place a left-sided chest drain in the left 4th intercostal space. Then, start a labetalol infusion in view of the widened mediastinum to maintain a systolic pressure of 100 mmHg and a pulse rate of around 60 bpm

D.   Rapid intubation and then perform a needle thoracostomy in the second intercostal space at the mid-clavicular line prior to arranging an urgent CT trauma of the chest, abdomen and pelvis

E.   Place bilateral chest drains and take to the angio suite for an urgent aortogram and placement of a thoracic endovascular stent graft for a likely blunt aortic injury

Q43. A 24-year-old man who suffered a severe head injury in a RTA 3 months earlier whilst under the influence of alcohol is to undergo brainstem death assessment in the intensive care unit. Which of the following statements is correct?

A.   The corneal reflex is elicited by touching the cornea with a piece of cotton wool. The corneal reflex tests cranial nerves III and V

B.   To perform the apnoea test, the patient is first given 100% oxygen to ensure adequate pre-oxygenation. Then, mechanical ventilation is physically disconnected and blood gas evaluations are taken every 5 minutes until $PaCO_2$ increases to 8.0 kPa or higher and pH <7.3. The test is considered positive if any signs of spontaneous respiration occur

C. Four-vessel cerebral angiography evaluating carotid and vertebral artery flow is widely considered the gold standard ancillary test when standard brainstem death tests are not possible to be performed

D. Before initiating brainstem tests, measure plasma levels of alcohol and ensure levels are not recordable

E. Three sets of brainstem death tests should be performed at separate time points by different doctors, one of whom must be involved in the transplant service

Q44. A 75-year-old man underwent a right femoral embolectomy earlier in the morning, and you are called in the early evening because he is now experiencing severe pain in his right calf. His calf is tender and his foot has no sensation and is cool to palpation. Based on this information, which of the following is most likely:

A. He has developed a haematoma in his right calf that is compressing his popliteal artery

B. He is developing compartment syndrome in his calf and needs an emergency three-compartment fasciotomy

C. He has continued to develop acute lower limb ischaemia either because his femoral artery has rethrombosed or he suffered distal embolisation into his calf arteries at the time of his embolectomy

D. The pain is likely related to ischaemic neuropathy, and the cool foot relates to an autonomic dysfunction

E. He may have suffered an embolic stroke following surgery

ANSWERS

Q1. Option C – Broad-spectrum intravenous antibiotic therapy only, discussing a significant risk of recurrence even if the treatment is successful

This is most likely uncomplicated appendicitis – Current evidence would support initial intravenous antibiotics. Patients should be informed that there is around a 40% recurrence rate at 5 years. Particularly, in a high-risk patient, a more conservative approach may be preferable. Thickening of the caecal pole is common in scan findings. If further investigations are required, these should be delayed until after the acute episode.

Q2. Option E – Intravenous co-amoxiclav with monitoring of clinical signs

Small pericolic abscesses can be treated with antibiotics initially and similarly isolated pericolic gas. Larger abscesses are less likely to respond to this treatment and percutaneous drainage should be considered. The antibiotic response may take 48 hours or more. A deterioration in condition would mandate urgent surgical exploration.

Q3. Option D – Uncomplicated stenting appears to be as oncologically safe at 3–5 years as emergency surgery

Q4. Option E – age > 70, blood pressure, digital rectal exam findings
　　　Oakland score comprises age, sex, previous lower GI bleed admission, digital rectal exam findings, heart rate, blood pressure and haemoglobin and gives a probability of re-admission. Hence, it allows an indication of what can be managed safely as an out-patient.

Q5. Option A – Laparoscopic cholecystectomy with on-table cholangiogram
　　　Given that there is no derangement of bilirubin, it should be safe to remove the gall bladder to prevent future attacks and relieve pain/inflammation/infection. Small stones found at cholangiography can be dealt with by CBD exploration laparoscopically of subsequent MRCP/ERCP – see the AUGIS guidelines for acute gallstone disease.

Q6. Option C – The anion gap is cut by 40%
　　　The rest are evidence-based observations

Q7. Option B – A 'swinging' arterial trace may indicate hypovolaemia
　　　Differing amplitudes during the respiratory cycle are described as 'swinging' and may indicate hypovolaemia

Q8. Option B – The infusion is placed deep into the ligamentum flavum
　　　A loss of resistance is felt on piercing the ligamentum flavum and indicates correct positioning

Q9. Option E – Laparotomy ileo-caecectomy and ileostomy
　　　Pseudo-obstruction with caecum > 12 cm, caecal tenderness and leukocytosis are highly likely to indicate caecal ischaemia from radial wall tension, and impending perforation. If the patient is fit enough, the colon requires surgical decompression and the caecum will need to be resected. Anastomosis is inadvisable given the pseudo-obstruction. An ileostomy and mucus fistula give the safest immediate outcome.

Q10. Option C – Transfer to a CT scanner for chest, abdomen and pelvis CT
　　　A fluid-responsive patient may be stabilised enough for a trauma series CT scan. This will give valuable diagnostic information to guide intervention and prioritisation of interventions.

Q11. Option D – 25–30 mL/kg/day water, 1 mmol/kg/day potassium, sodium and chloride, and 50–100 g/day glucose
　　　The principles are to avoid hyperchloraemic acidosis and avoid starvation ketosis

Q12. Option A – CT scan of the abdomen and pelvis
　　　In this case, the fact that the patient has a high BMI and had a bariatric operation leads to the differential diagnosis of internal hernia or biliary colic. RYGB's early or late complication can be the internal hernia. Even though laparoscopy is

an option, the most appropriate next step is to request a CT scan of the abdomen and pelvis. This will exclude the internal hernia that can be catastrophic however in circumstances of high suspicion we would still laparoscope. Gastroscopy is not a good option at this stage. An ultrasound scan can exclude cholelithiasis; however, its diagnostic value is limited in obese patients.

Q13. Option C – CT scan of the pelvis

In this case, an obese diabetic patient with recurrent perianal abscesses and a presentation in A&E with sepsis most likely have a recurrence of a complex perianal abscess. However, necrotising fasciitis should be excluded as it can be lethal. CT scan of the pelvis will help with diagnostics in this case and then of course exploration with incision and drainage plus minus proceed will be the next step. MRI of the pelvis cannot/is challenging in an emergency situation with a septic patient. Antibiotics should be given straight away; however, conservative management should be decided after appropriate imaging and appropriate clinical context.

Q14. Option E – Diagnostic laparoscopy

The mechanism of injury indicated that there is a high-impact collision in the abdominal area of the patient. Most common injuries in that area involve the pancreas, the vessels, the bowel, the stomach, the spleen or the liver. The CT scan of the abdomen and pelvis excluded a liver, vascular, pancreatic and spleen injury. However, a CT scan cannot exclude a bowel or gastric injury/perforation. WBCs are quite high, and this indicates intrabdominal infection. The finding of fluid with FAST scan and CT scan is alerting. Diagnostic laparoscopy is the next appropriate step as this will exclude a bowel or gastric injury/perforation and reveal the type of intrabdominal fluid. Diagnostic laparotomy is more invasive and has no benefit in this case compared with the laparoscopic approach. A repeat of the CT scan will not facilitate the diagnosis in case of a bowel or gastric injury and within 24 hours the patient may be unwell or unstable to move to the scanner. A repeat of the FAST scan is a good option but will help the diagnosis only if there is significantly more fluid in the abdomen. A repeat of blood tests can be requested for the review but will not actually facilitate the diagnosis.

Q15. Option E – Pack the rectum with gauze

This patient is 88 and unstable. She is not suitable for CT angiogram; however, it seems that the bleeding is diffuse from the rectum and anus (radiation-related). Close observation and transfuse are acceptable, but the patient is bleeding actively and this needs to be addressed as soon as possible. Flexible sigmoidoscopy is not appropriate in this phase as the patient is unstable and it will not add anything to the management. EUA±proceed will be risky as the patient is unstable and frail, possibly not fit for general anaesthetic. Stopping the bleeding with aggressive packing of the rectum is the first course of action in order to limit the blood loss and give some time for the patient to recover with a combination of transfusion and TXA. There is more current evidence however that TXA is more appropriately used in trauma rather than in other bleeding scenarios.

Q16. Option D – CT scan of the abdomen and pelvis

The mechanism of injury, the use of anticoagulation, and the low Hgb and BP show the presence of bleeding. The rigidness of the abdomen is a surgical emergency and requires an early aggressive intervention which most of the time is an exploratory laparotomy. However, in this case, there is a high possibility of rectus sheath haematoma which can cause rigidity of the abdomen, but laparotomy is not always the indicated treatment option. Hence, in this case, we will proceed with imaging to obtain some more information and decide then for further management.

Q17. Option D – Change to intravenous antibiotic and arrange urgent debridement

Necrotising fasciitis (NF) is a rare but life-threatening condition affecting the soft tissues and fascia. NF is usually the result of a recent skin break (such as trauma, or surgery), which allows pathogens to enter the soft tissues. NF can be divided into four types: Type I (polymicrobial), type 2 (Streptococcus), type III (gas gangrene) and other types (e.g., due to fungi). The prognosis is poor, with up to a third of patients with NF dying from infection.

Symptoms of NF progress from disproportionate pain and fever in the early stages to progressive necrosis, sepsis and toxic shock. Diagnosis is generally clinical (i.e. through a high index of suspicion and patient assessment). Early, aggressive treatment is essential.

In 2014, the World Society of Emergency Surgery (WSES) published guidelines for the management of skin and soft tissue infections, which encompasses NF. For all necrotising soft tissue infections, early appropriate empiric antimicrobial therapy should be given. In cases of necrotising infection associated with severe sepsis or septic shock, early source control is advised; this is in the form of aggressive surgical debridement.

Q18. Option D – Admission for surgery during the night

This scenario reflects a patient with a strangulated hernia containing small bowel which is at risk of irreversible ischaemia.

In 2017, the World Society of Emergency Surgery (WSES) published guidelines for the emergency repair of complicated abdominal wall hernias. They recommend immediate hernia repair if intestinal strangulation is suspected.

The National Confidential Enquiry into Patient Outcome and Death (NCEPOD) categorise the urgency of an operation into immediate, urgent, expedited and elective according to the risk to the patient. In this classification, the above patient would be deemed "urgent" (i.e. acute onset or deterioration that threatens life, limb or organ survival) and thereby has a target time to theatre within hours of the decision to operate.

Q19. Option C – *Helicobacter pylori* infection

Peptic ulcers are common, with a lifetime prevalence of 5%–10%. The incidence of duodenal ulcers peaks at 45–64 years, whereas the incidence of gastric ulcers increases with age. Duodenal ulcers are more common in men. The most common risk factors for duodenal ulcers are *H. pylori* infection (approximately 90%) and NSAID/aspirin (approximately 10%); other rare causes include SSRIs, smoking, Zollinger Ellison syndrome, physiological stress, tumours and autoimmune disease. The management of uncomplicated peptic ulcers is acid suppression with PPI and treatment/elimination of risk factors. Whilst in a small subgroup of patients non-operative management may be appropriate, surgery remains the mainstay of treatment for ulcer perforation.

Q20. Option C – CT with arterial contrast

Acute mesenteric ischaemia (AMI) is a rare cause of abdominal pain but is associated with a high mortality rate and so early diagnosis and intervention are both essential. The causes of AMI can be divided into non-occlusive or occlusive, with occlusive further sub-divided into mesenteric arterial embolism, mesenteric arterial thrombosis or mesenteric venous thrombosis. Acute mesenteric arterial embolism is the most common cause of AMI (approximately 50%), with the most common site of occlusion being the superior mesenteric artery. Acute mesenteric arterial thrombosis (25% AMI) is generally found in patients with pre-existing atherosclerosis/stenosis; acute mesenteric venous thrombosis (<10% AMI) is secondary to hyper-coagulopathic tendency. Non-occlusive ischaemia is secondary to reduced blood flow to the mesenteric vessels, such as with a critical illness, cardiac failure or vasoconstrictors.

Most commonly patients present with severe abdominal pain disproportionate to clinical findings, often accompanied by nausea, vomiting, and/or diarrhoea. Later features (suggesting intestinal infarction) include peritonitis, bloody diarrhoea and shock. The World Society for Emergency Surgery (WSES) recommends that "severe abdominal pain out of proportion to physical examination findings should be assumed to be AMI until disproven".

For any patient with suspected AMI, it is recommended that CT angiography should be performed as soon as possible. Treatment of AMI includes resuscitation, antibiotics, resection of any necrotic bowel and revascularisation/reperfusion.

Q21. Option C – CT abdomen with contrast

The overall risk of perforation following colonoscopy is approximately 0.07%, with around 50% with a perforation requiring surgery. The risk of perforation for therapeutic colonoscopy (including polypectomy) is higher at 0.1%, with the main risk factors for perforation being the size and location of the polyps (higher risk more proximally). Approximately half of the iatrogenic colonic perforations are identified by the endoscopist at the time of the procedure.

The most common presentation of colonic perforation detected after colonoscopy is abdominal pain within 48 hours of the procedure, although symptoms and findings can be variable depending on the size of the perforation, location, and amount of contamination. Whilst plain X-ray has a high positive predictive value, it is not sensitive, so in any patient where there is suspicion of colonoscopic perforation, a CT with contrast should be performed.

The treatment of post-colonoscopic perforations may be conservative, endoscopic or surgical. Factors favouring a conservative approach are haemodynamic stability and absence of sepsis, generalised pain, or free fluid; endoscopic therapy may be considered within 4 hours of the perforation if it is small and if there is available expertise/experience. If there is peritonism, sepsis, suspicion of a large perforation or poor bowel preparation, then surgery is indicated, and, likewise, in cases of failed conservative management or underlying bowel pathology.

Q22. Option D – diversion colostomy

Following the extensive literature review, the Eastern Association for the Surgery of Trauma produced guidelines for the management of penetrating extraperitoneal rectal injuries, published in 2016. These guidelines focus on low-velocity, non-destructive injuries (i.e. <25% circumference). Specifically, the guidelines are for extraperitoneal injuries, recommending that intraperitoneal rectal injuries are managed like colonic injuries. These guidelines advise against the use of rectal washouts or drains due to a lack of evidence. Although the quality of evidence was deemed low, the proximal colonic diversion was recommended, as in previous studies, it halved the risk of infectious complications.

Q23. Option D – Ultrasound-guided aspiration±culture

Principles of management of breast infections:

- Antibiotics should be given early to reduce the risk of developing breast abscesses
  - If the infection does not settle within 48 hours with antibiotics treatment, hospital referral is indicated
  - If an abscess is suspected, an ultrasound scan should be performed to confirm its presence before any drainage is attempted
  - Breast cancer should be excluded in patients with a solid mass on USS or does not settle despite sufficient antibiotic therapy
    Predisposing factors for breast abscess in non-lactational women:
  - Smoking: Nicotine and toxins accumulate in the breasts causing local hypoxic damage to the ducts.
  - Nipple damage: caused by piercing, eczema, infection or Raynaud's disease can be a source of bacterial entry.
  - Breast abnormalities: Ductal abnormalities, cysts and tumours can cause persistent poor drainage, leading to infection.
  - Other factors such as immunosuppression, foreign bodies (i.e. silicone) and shaving of the areolar hair can lead to breast infection.
    The presence of a tender swelling and erythema suggests an abscess. Breast abscesses are best treated with Ultrasound-guided aspiration followed by culture to guide further antibiotic therapy. Aspiration can be repeated every 2–3 days if a recollection has happened.

If surgical drainage is needed a small incision (<1 cm) should be used to allow the pus to drain, and no packing should be performed as there is enough evidence that it will delay the healing.

Q24. Option B – Urgent CT

Acute appendicitis is a common cause of acute abdomen. Imaging modalities are used to guide the diagnosis and to avoid negative appendicectomy, the rate of which can reach up to 15%.

Differential diagnoses include acute appendicitis, appendicular mass and ileocolic Crohn's disease. Often the diagnosis of appendicitis is clinical; however, in cases where there is diagnostic uncertainty (particularly in a stable patient), then imaging should be performed. In this case, an urgent CT with contrast should be performed to guide further treatment.

Abdominal USS is cost-effective, harmless and useful in assessing pelvic organs in females; however, it is user-dependent and has lower sensitivity when compared to a CT scan in diagnosing acute appendicitis (76% vs 94%).

Diagnostic laparoscopy might be performed if there is a lack of imaging techniques and diagnostic uncertainty.

Q25. Option E – CT with arterial contrast

In 2019, the BSG published guidelines on the management of lower GI bleeding, which categorised patients as stable or unstable according to their shock index (calculated by heart rate/systolic blood pressure). For stable patients, a luminal examination is recommended (either as an in-patient or out-patient), whereas unstable patients should undergo CT angiography initially. If on the CT angiogram extravasation of the contrast is detected, embolisation of the mesenteric vessel might be performed. If unable to control bleeding and if the patient remains unstable, then surgery should be considered (targeted at the localised bleeding point).

Q26. Option A – EUA and incision and drainage

The presence of a tender swelling is suggestive of a perianal abscess. The cryptoglandular theory of abscess formation is:

Obstruction of the anal crypts glands leads to infection and the formation of anorectal abscesses. It can be related to aerobics (*Staphylococcus aureus*, Streptococcus, Enterobacteriaceae and Enterococcus) or anaerobes (Bacteroides, Peptostreptococcus and Clostridium).

Most common types (Parks classification):

Inter-sphincteric 70% [between both sphincters]

Trans-sphincteric 25% [through both]

Supra-sphincteric 4% [above external then through internal]

Extra-sphincteric 1% [above both from outside]

This patient has Crohn's disease, suggesting that the abscess may be complex and there may be an associated fistula. Perianal abscesses secondary to Crohn's disease are generally difficult to treat, but in the acute setting, drainage of the abscess remains the priority.

Q27. Option B – Hartmann's procedure

Diverticular disease is a common disease in the western population with a lifetime risk of 4%. Management of Hinchey 3 diverticulitis (generalised purulent peritonitis) has been a topic of debate over the past few years. Laparoscopic lavage has been an acceptable practice following promising results from the DILALA trial in 2011; however, the recent termination of the LOLA arm of the LADIES trial due to a long-term increase in morbidity and mortality when compared to Hartmann's procedure has shifted most surgeons away from performing laparoscopic lavages. The WSES guidelines 2020 and the ACPGBI consensus guidelines have preserved the use of laparoscopic lavage in very few selected cases. In this case, the patient has multiple comorbidities, and is on inotropic support, making any anastomosis high risk.

Q28. Option E – Right hemicolectomy

Colonic volvulus is a general surgical emergency, it usually presents with abdominal pain, distention, and nausea. Sigmoid volvulus is common in males, whilst caecal volvulus is common in females. Two to 5% causes of large bowel obstruction are caused by volvulus.

A large study from the United States has investigated the outcomes of colonic volvulus, in which resection in caecal volvulus has a better outcome than caecopexy. Small case series have reported a high success rate for percutaneous caecostomy, it should be preserved for high-risk patients as there is reported high morbidity and mortality in the literature.

The ACPGBI consensus in emergency colorectal surgery which was published in 2020 recommends surgical resection for caecal volvulus.

Although an NG tube will decompress the GI tract and potentially improve the patient's symptoms and allow for better electrolyte management, it is not the definitive management in this case. Gastrograffin is primarily in cases of small bowel obstruction due to adhesional cause. Endoscopic detorsion is usually effective in managing sigmoid volvulus; however, it has a low success rate in caecal volvulus.

Q29. Option C – 10%–20%

Ulcerative colitis (UC) is one of the two large types of inflammatory bowel disease, the other being Crohn's disease. It is a disease of the Western world with an incidence rate between 2 and 15/100,000. It is less prevalent in Asia, Africa, South America, and South-eastern Europe. It has a near-equal predominance in both females and males.

Truelove and Witts classification has been developed in 1954. It classifies acute colitis into mild, moderate and severe to guide the management of patients at the acute presentation. It includes a number of motions per day and the presence of blood, as well as systematic features such as ESR, anaemia and the presence of pyrexia.

The majority of acute admissions can be satisfactorily managed with medical therapy, and around 30%–40% will require colectomy at some point. Ten to twenty per cent of patients with acute severe UC will need surgical resection on their first admission.

Q30. Option D – Boerhaave's syndrome

Boerhaave syndrome is also known as spontaneous oesophageal rupture or effort rupture of the oesophagus. Although vomiting is thought to be the most common cause, other causes include those that can increase intra-oesophagal pressure and cause a barogenic oesophageal rupture. The disorder may present with vague symptoms, or one may note the classic Mackler triad of vomiting, chest pain, and subcutaneous emphysema. Imaging examination is of great significance for the early diagnosis of Boerhaave's syndrome. Chest radiology examination findings such as pleural effusion or pneumomediastinum are of great significance for diagnosis. Thoracic CT is helpful in differential diagnosis with other traumatic oesophageal injuries. Further contrast oesophagography may provide exact evidence of contrast leakage from the oesophageal lumen to make a definite diagnosis. The mainstay of treatment includes volume replacement, broad-spectrum antibiotic coverage and surgical evaluation. Surgical intervention includes primary oesophageal repair through open thoracotomy vs. VATS or T-tube drainage, which is the gold standard within the first 24 hours. Endoscopic placement of stents has been used to prevent fistula formations or seal oesophageal leaks both in patients with delayed diagnoses and those with early diagnoses without widespread contamination. Conservative measurements are usually reserved for small or contained ruptures.

Q31. Option C – Open conversion and liver packing

Approximately 0.1%–2.0% of cases have uncontrolled bleeding during laparoscopic cholecystectomy, and around 80% of them are from the gall-bladder bed. Bleeding from the middle hepatic vein may result in cases where the vein is directly exposed or adhered to the gall-bladder bed which is around 10% of cases.

Q32. Option D – Pancreatic pseudocyst

A pancreatic pseudocyst is a type of cyst that is not contained inside an enclosed sac of its own with an epithelium lining. Instead, the pseudocyst forms within a cavity or space inside the pancreas and is surrounded by fibrous tissue. Pancreatic pseudocysts do contain inflammatory pancreatic fluid (particularly the digestive enzyme amylase) or semisolid matter. A pseudocyst is formed following an episode of acute pancreatitis, often within 4–6 weeks of that episode, with a well-defined wall lined by granulation or fibrous tissue. The most common symptoms include severe, persistent pain in the abdomen and sometimes the back, nausea, vomiting and abdominal bloating.

Q33. Option A – Washout plus Subhepatic wide-bore drain

Bile leakage is an uncommon complication of cholecystectomy. The bile may originate from the gall-bladder bed, the cystic duct or from injury to a bile duct. Although a CT scan can be performed in the first instance in stable patients, its sensitivity and specificity are not 100% to pick up bile duct injury/bile leak and so clinical suspicion should remain high in any patient with significant pain following cholecystectomy. The primary goal of treatment is drainage of intraperitoneal bile, and control of any ongoing leak via drains; whilst this may be possible with interventional radiology in selected cases, the most common method is laparoscopy. Once the patient has stabilised and the leak is controlled, the investigation into the cause may be considered, with subsequent treatment as necessary.

Q34. Option C – Laparoscopic cholecystectomy + intraoperative cholangiogram

Traumatic gall-bladder rupture occurs rarely and the incidence is reported to amount to approximately 2% of all blunt abdominal injuries. The main reason for the low incidence is that the gall bladder is protected by the surrounding organs, including the liver, intestines, omentum, and ribs. In stable patients, laparoscopy instead of laparotomy is being attempted more often, especially in isolated organ injuries. There can be a concomitant injury to bile ducts and IOC will reveal not only those but also confirm the anatomy before dividing the cystic duct and artery to perform cholecystectomy. This is furthermore important medico legally as pre-existing bile duct injuries due to trauma (and not operative intervention) will be revealed

Q35. Option C – 30%–40% circulating volume

Shock is defined as inadequate organ perfusion and tissue oxygenation due to an abnormality of the circulatory system. Hypovolemia is the cause of shock in most trauma patients. Treatment requires rapid haemorrhage control and fluid resuscitation with fluid and/or blood products.

The DDx of shock is either haemorrhagic or non-haemorrhagic. Causes of non-haemorrhagic shock are:

- Cardiogenic
- Cardiac tamponade
- Tension pneumothorax
- Neurogenic
- Septic

Haemorrhagic shock can be classified into four classes based on clinical signs and symptoms which can be used for predicting estimated blood loss which in turn can be used to guide treatment; ATLS categorised these into classes 1–4, which correspond to blood loss of 15% (750 mL approx.), 15%–30% (750–1,500 mL), 30%–40% (1,500–2,000 mL approx.) and >40% (>2,000 mL approx.), respectively. In this case, the patient has class 3 shock, equating to 30%–40% blood loss.

Careful response to fluid resuscitation should be used with 'permissive hypotension' currently advocated.

Q36. Option D – In-patient OGD with banding of varices

Variceal haemorrhage is defined as bleeding from an oesophageal or gastric varix. An episode of bleeding is clinically significant when there is a transfusion requirement for 2 units of blood in 24 hours from presentation, with <100 mmHg or >100 bpm.

OGD should be done in unstable patients immediately after resuscitation. All other patients with UGI bleeding should be offered endoscopy within 24 hours of admission.

Antibiotics are recommended for all patients with variceal bleeding. Band ligation is recommended as the preferred endoscopic method. Proton pump inhibitors are not recommended unless otherwise required. Vasoconstrictors (terlipressin or somatostatin) are recommended and be continued until haemostasis is achieved. After haemostasis, TIPSS can be considered

If bleeding is difficult to control, a Sengstaken–Blakemore tube should be inserted until further endoscopic treatment, TIPSS or surgery is performed depending on local resources and expertise.

Q37. Option B – Wide-bore NG tube insertion bedside

The description from the CT scan is that of organoaxial gastric volvulus. Acute gastric volvulus classically presents with Borchardt's triad; severe epigastric pain, vomiting, and difficulty or inability to pass a nasogastric tube. There is a risk of progression to gastric ischaemia which in turn can lead to perforation. Chronically, it can present vaguely with dysphagia, pain, bloating, nausea and vomiting, dyspepsia and shortness of breath.

Initial management involves resuscitation, blood, NGT (by an experienced person and imagining CT CAP in the acute setting±oral contrast). If there is gastric necrosis or perforation, or the patient is acutely unwell, surgical repair must be considered. If stable, you can consider OGD±laparoscopy to aid decompression. Conservative management can be trialled in healthy patients with no concerning findings on CT and decompression has been achieved with NGT.

Q38. Option A – Admission for observation

This patient would have a WSES grade I injury (AAST grade II) and be classified as a minor injury by the WSES 2020 guidelines. Given that the patient is haemodynamically stable with a minor injury and no blush sign, they should be admitted for observation and serial investigation/imaging. Embolisation could be considered with this level of injury if there was an arterial blush sign on the CT scan. An absolute requirement for non-operative management is haemodynamic stability and the absence of other lesions requiring surgery, and this is true of blunt and penetrating trauma of the liver.

Q39. Option D

NF is a life-threatening condition and will require urgent and aggressive surgical debridement to gain source control. This patient's observations do not meet the criteria for sepsis based on qSOFA score which includes respiratory rate $\geq$22, altered mentation (GCS < 15) and systolic BP < 100 mmHg. However, instigating the sepsis 6 bundle is appropriate.

Q40. Option C

Anuria should prompt a clinician to consider a urinary outflow problem such as a blocked urinary catheter. This is the most likely diagnosis in this case. Lower abdominal pain relates to a distended bladder. He has nothing in his history or vital signs that would raise suspicion of ureteric injury or anastomotic leak. Bilateral ureteric injury is very unlikely and would present much earlier. Pre-renal failure from hypovolaemia can eventually result in anuria but oliguria would be recorded for a longer period of time first.

Q41. Option B

Hyperkalaemia of 6.9 mmol/L is immediately life-threatening. Initial treatment should involve calcium gluconate for cardiac protection, particularly given the widened QRS complexes. It also involves shifting K+ from extracellular to intracellular by means of dextrose/insulin and using salbutamol. Treatments such as calcium resonium will take longer to have an effect. The patient is likely to require RRT, but it is important to reduce K+ quicker to prevent a life-threatening arrhythmia.

Q42. Option B

This patient should be considered to have a blunt thoracic aortic injury in addition to a large pneumothorax. The history is a classic acceleration–deceleration trauma scenario. Following chest drain insertion, the diagnosis of a blunt thoracic aortic injury is best made with a CT angiogram. This can be part of a standard CT trauma sequence. The management of these injuries is by thoracic endovascular stent grafts deployed through the femoral arteries. It is good practice to maintain a permissive hypotensive approach to resuscitation until the aortic injury is treated, but in a trauma situation, it is unlikely that reduced impulse therapy such as labetalol infusion is required or appropriate.

Q43. Option C

The brainstem tests should be repeated on two occasions once any reversible causes for coma and apnoea have been excluded and no doctor with a conflict of interest; e.g., the transplant surgeon should be involved. In relation to alcohol, the levels should be below the legal limit for driving. Corneal reflex test cranial nerves V and VII. The apnoea test is considered positive if there are no signs of spontaneous respiration are recorded.

Q44. Option C

Pain in the calf after femoral embolectomy can be a sign of compartment syndrome, but the fact that the calf was tender and the foot is cool is more likely to be related to ongoing ischaemia with muscle necrosis, causing the calf tenderness. Compartment syndrome tends to cause a swollen warm leg from successful reperfusion with tenderness in the calf.

FURTHER READING

American College of Surgeons. Advanced Trauma Life Support: Student Course Manual. Tenth ed. Chicago, IL: American College of Surgeons; 2018.

Aratari A, Papi C, Clemente V, Moretti A, Luchetti R, Koch M, Capurso L, Caprilli R. Colectomy rate in acute severe ulcerative colitis in the infliximab era. *Dig Liver Dis.* 2008 Oct;40(10):821–826. doi: 10.1016/j.dld.2008.03.014.

Bala M, et al. Acute mesenteric ischemia: guidelines of the World Society of Emergency Surgery. *World J Emerg Surg.* 2017 Aug 7;12:38. doi: 10.1186/s13017-017-0150-5.

Ball CG, MacLean AR, Kirkpatrick AW, Bathe OF, Sutherland F, et al. Hepatic vein injury during laparoscopic cholecystectomy: the unappreciated proximity of the middle hepatic vein to the gallbladder bed. *J Gastrointest Surg.* 2006;10:1151–1155.

Banks PA, Bollen TL, Dervenis C, Gooszen HG, Johnson CD, Sarr MG, Tsiotos GG, Vege SS. Acute Pancreatitis Classification Working Group. Classification of acute pancreatitis–2012: revision of the Atlanta classification and definitions by international consensus. *Gut.* 2013 Jan;62(1):102–111.

Birindelli A, et al. 2017 update of the WSES guidelines for emergency repair of complicated abdominal wall hernias. *World J Emerg Surg.* 2017 Aug 7;12:37. doi: 10.1186/s13017-017-0149-y.

Bolkenstein HE, van Dijk ST, Consten ECJ, Heggelman BGF, Hoeks CMA, Broeders IAMJ, Boermeester MA, Draaisma WA. Conservative treatment in diverticulitis patients with pericolic extraluminal air and the role of antibiotic treatment. *J Gastrointest Surg.* 2019 Nov;23(11):2269–2276. doi: 10.1007/s11605-019-04153-9.

Bosarge PL, et al. Management of penetrating extraperitoneal rectal injuries. *J Trauma Acute Care Surg.* 2016;80(3):546–551. doi: 10.1097/TA.0000000000000953.

Centers for Disease Control and Prevention. *Necrotizing fasciitis.* CDC. 2019. Available at: https://www.cdc.gov/groupastrep/diseases-public/necrotizingfasciitis.html (Accessed: May 22nd, 2022).

Coccolini F, Coimbra R, Ordonez C, et al. Liver trauma: WSES 2020 guidelines. *World J Emerg Surg.* 2020;15:24. doi: 10.1186/s13017-020-00302-7.

De'Angelis N, Catena F, Memeo R, et al. 2020 WSES guidelines for the detection and management of bile duct injury during cholecystectomy. *World J Emerg Surg.* 2021;16:30. doi: 10.1186/s13017-021-00369-w.

de'Angelis N, et al. 2017 WSES guidelines for the management of iatrogenic colonoscopy perforation. *World J Emerg Surg.* 2018 Jan 24;13:5. doi: 10.1186/s13017-018-0162-9.

Dinesen LC, Walsh AJ, Protic MN, Heap G, Cummings F, Warren BF, George B, Mortensen NJ, Travis SP. The pattern and outcome of acute severe colitis. *J Crohns Colitis*. 2010 Oct;4(4):431–437. doi: 10.1016/j.crohns.2010.02.001.

Gingold D, Murrell Z. Management of colonic volvulus. *Clin Colon Rectal Surg*. 2012 Dec;25(4):236–244. doi: 10.1055/s-0032-1329535.

Gorter, R.R., Eker, H.H., Gorter-Stam, M.A.W. et al. Diagnosis and management of acute appendicitis. EAES consensus development conference 2015. *Surg Endosc*. 2016;(11):4668–4690.

Gosselink MP, van Onkelen RS, Schouten WR. The cryptoglandular theory revisited. *Colorectal Dis*. 2015 Dec;17(12):1041–1043. doi: 10.1111/codi.13161.

Halabi WJ, Jafari MD, Kang CY, Nguyen VQ, Carmichael JC, Mills S, Pigazzi A, Stamos MJ. Colonic volvulus in the United States: trends, outcomes, and predictors of mortality. *Ann Surg*. 2014 Feb;259(2):293–301. doi: 10.1097/SLA.0b013e31828c88ac.

Hauge T, Kleven OC, Johnson E, Hofstad B, Johannessen HO. Outcome after stenting and débridement for spontaneous oesophagal rupture. *Scand J Gastroenterol*. 2018 Apr;53(4):398–402.

https://members.augis.org/Portals/0/Guidelines/Acute-Gallstones-Pathway-Final-Sept-2015.pdf?ver=8SLL3_E_X7VSx4gqyVYd6Q%3d%3d

https://www.nice.org.uk/guidance/ng39/chapter/recommendations

Hunter Lanier M, Ludwig DR, Ilahi O, Mellnick V. Prognostic value of water-soluble contrast challenge for nonadhesive small bowel obstruction. *J Am Coll Surg*. 2022 Feb 1;234(2):121–128. doi: 10.1097/XCS.0000000000000020.

Kougias P, Lau D, El Sayed HF, Zhou W, Huynh TT, Lin PH. Determinants of mortality and treatment outcome following surgical interventions for acute mesenteric ischemia. *J Vasc Surg*. 2007 Sep;46(3): 467–474.

Lam E, Chan T, Wiseman SM. Breast abscess: evidence based management recommendations. *Expert Rev Anti Infect Ther*. 2014 Jul;12(7):753–762. doi: 10.1586/14787210.2014.913982.

Lambrichts DPV, Vennix S, Musters GD, Mulder IM, Swank HA, Hoofwijk AGM, Belgers EHJ, Stockmann HBAC, Eijsbouts QAJ, Gerhards MF, van Wagensveld BA, van Geloven AAW, Crolla RMPH, Nienhuijs SW, Govaert MJPM, di Saverio S, D'Hoore AJL, Consten ECJ, van Grevenstein WMU, Pierik REGJM, Kruyt PM, van der Hoeven JAB, Steup WH, Catena F, Konsten JLM, Vermeulen J, van Dieren S, Bemelman WA, Lange JF; LADIES trial collaborators. Hartmann's procedure versus sigmoidectomy with primary anastomosis for perforated diverticulitis with purulent or faecal peritonitis (LADIES): a multicentre, parallel-group, randomised, open-label, superiority trial. *Lancet Gastroenterol Hepatol*. 2019 Aug;4(8):599–610. doi: 10.1016/S2468-1253(19)30174-8.

Lameris W, van Randen A, van Es HW, et al. Imaging strategies for detection of urgent conditions in patients with acute abdominal pain: diagnostic accuracy study. *BMJ*. 2009;338:b2431.

Lanas A, Chan FKL. Peptic ulcer disease. *Lancet*. 2017;6736(16):1–12.

Light D, Links D, Griffin M. The threatened stomach: management of the acute gastric volvulus. *Surg Endosc*. 2016 May;30(5):1847–1852. doi: 10.1007/s00464-015-4425-1.

Lynch CR, Jones RG, Hilden K, Wills JC, Fang JC. Percutaneous endoscopic cecostomy in adults: a case series. *Gastrointest Endosc*. 2006 Aug;64(2):279–282. doi: 10.1016/j.gie.2006.02.037.

Miller AS, Boyce K, Box B, Clarke MD, Duff SE, Foley NM, Guy RJ, Massey LH, Ramsay G, Slade DAJ, Stephenson JA, Tozer PJ, Wright D. The Association of Coloproctology of Great Britain and Ireland consensus guidelines in emergency colorectal surgery. *Colorectal Dis*. 2021 Feb;23(2):476–547. doi: 10.1111/codi.15503.

National Confidential Enquiry into Patient Outcome and Death. *The NCEPOD classification of intervention*. NCEPOD. 2004. Available at: https://www.ncepod.org.uk/classification.html (Accessed: May 22nd, 2022).

National Institute for Health and Care Excellence. *Dyspepsia – Proven peptic ulcer: What are the risk factors?* NICE. 2019. Available at: https://cks.nice.org.uk/topics/dyspepsia-proven-peptic-ulcer/background-information/risk-factors/ (Accessed: May 22nd, 2022)

Naveed M, Jamil LH, Fujii-Lau LL, Al-Haddad M, Buxbaum JL, Fishman DS, Jue TL, Law JK, Lee JK, Qumseya BJ, Sawhney MS, Thosani N, Storm AC, Calderwood AH, Khashab MA, Wani SB. American Society for Gastrointestinal Endoscopy guideline on the role of endoscopy in the management of acute colonic pseudo-obstruction and colonic volvulus. *Gastrointest Endosc*. 2020 Feb;91(2):228–235. doi: 10.1016/j.gie.2019.09.007. Erratum in: *Gastrointest Endosc*. 2020 Mar;91(3):721.

Newman J, Fitzgerald JE, Gupta S, von Roon AC, Sigurdsson HH, Allen-Mersh TG. Outcome predictors in acute surgical admissions for lower gastrointestinal bleeding. *Colorectal Dis*. 2012 Aug;14(8):1020–1026. doi: 10.1111/j.1463-1318.2011.02824.x.

Ngan V, Gomez J. *Necrotising fasciitis*. Dermnet NZ. 2016. Available at: https://dermnetnz.org/topics/necrotising-fasciitis (Accessed: May 22nd, 2022).

NICE Clinical Guideline CG174. Intravenous Fluid Therapy in Adults in Hospital. 2013.

Oakland K, Guy R, Uberoi R, et al. Acute lower GI bleeding in the UK: patient characteristics, interventions and outcomes in the first nationwide audit. *Gut*. 2018;67:654–662.

Okamoto H, Onodera K, Kamba R, Taniyama Y, Sakurai T, Heishi T, Teshima J, Hikage M, Sato C, Maruyama S, Onodera Y, Ishida H, Kamei T. Treatment of spontaneous esophageal rupture (Boerhaave syndrome) using thoracoscopic surgery and sivelestat sodium hydrate. *J Thorac Dis*. 2018 Apr;10(4):2206–2212.

Panteris V, Haringsma J, Kuipers EJ. Colonoscopy perforation rate, mechanisms and outcome: from diagnostic to therapeutic colonoscopy. *Endoscopy*. 2009;41:941–951.

Parks AG, Gordon PH, Hardcastle JD. A classification of fistula-in-ano. *Br J Surg*. 1976 Jan;63(1):1–12. doi: 10.1002/bjs.1800630102.

Public Health England. *Bowel cancer screening: having a colonoscopy*. Gov.UK. 2021. Available at: https://www.gov.uk/government/publications/bowel-cancer-screening-colonoscopy/bowel-cancer-screening-having-a-colonoscopy-fit (Accessed: May 22nd, 2022).

Public Health England. *Guidance: Necrotising fasciitis*. Gov.UK. 2013. Available at: https://www.gov.uk/guidance/necrotising-fasciitis-nf (Accessed: May 22nd, 2022).

Rees CJ, Thomas Gibson S, Rutter MD, et al. UK key performance indicators and quality assurance standards for colonoscopy. *Gut*. 2016 Dec;65(12):1923–1929. doi: 10.1136/gutjnl-2016-312044.

Rutter MD, et al. Risk factors for adverse events related to polypectomy in the English Bowel Cancer Screening Programme. *Endoscopy*. 2014;46:90–97.

Sala E, Watson CJ, Beadsmoore C, et al. A randomized, controlled trial of routine early abdominal computed tomography in patients presenting with non-specific acute abdominal pain. *Clin Radiol*. 2007;62(10):961–969.

Salminen P, Tuominen R, Paajanen H, Rautio T, Nordström P, Aarnio M, Rantanen T, Hurme S, Mecklin JP, Sand J, Virtanen J, Jartti A, Grönroos JM. Five-year follow-up of antibiotic therapy for uncomplicated acute appendicitis in the APPAC randomized clinical trial. *JAMA*. 2018 Sep 25;320(12):1259–1265. doi: 10.1001/jama.2018.13201.

Sartelli M, et al. World Society of Emergency Surgery (WSES) guidelines for management of skin and soft tissue infections. *World J Emerg Surg*. 2014 Nov 18;9(1):57. doi: 10.1186/1749-7922-9-57.

Sartelli M, Weber DG, Kluger Y, Ansaloni L, Coccolini F, Abu-Zidan F, Augustin G, Ben-Ishay O, Biffl WL, Bouliaris K, Catena R, Ceresoli M, Chiara O, Chiarugi M, Coimbra R, Cortese F, Cui Y, Damaskos D, De'Angelis GL, Delibegovic S, Demetrashvili Z, De Simone B, Di Marzo F, Di Saverio S, Duane TM, Faro MP, Fraga GP, Gkiokas G, Gomes CA, Hardcastle TC, Hecker A, Karamarkovic A, Kashuk J, Khokha V, Kirkpatrick AW, Kok KYY, Inaba K, Isik A, Labricciosa FM, Latifi R, Leppäniemi A, Litvin A, Mazuski JE, Maier RV, Marwah S, McFarlane M, Moore EE, Moore FA, Negoi I, Pagani L, Rasa K, Rubio-Perez I, Sakakushev B, Sato N, Sganga G, Siquini W, Tarasconi A, Tolonen M, Ulrych J, Zachariah SK, Catena F. 2020 update of the WSES guidelines for the management of acute colonic diverticulitis in the emergency setting. *World J Emerg Surg*. 2020 May 7;15(1):32. doi: 10.1186/s13017-020-00313-4.

Scenario: Management – breast abscess | Management | Mastitis and breast abscess | CKS | NICE [Internet]. Available from: https://cks.nice.org.uk/topics/mastitis-breast-abscess/management/management-breast-abscess/

Shahedi K, Fuller G, Bolus R, Cohen E, Vu M, Shah R, et al. Long-term risk of acute diverticulitis among patients with incidental diverticulosis found during colonoscopy. *Clin Gastroenterol Hepatol*. 2013;11:1609–1613.

Sharma O. Blunt gallbladder injuries: presentation of twenty-two cases with review of the literature. *J Trauma*. 1995;39:576–580.

Soderstrom CA, Maekawa K, DuPriest RW Jr, Cowley RA. Gallbladder injuries resulting from blunt abdominal trauma: an experience and review. *Ann Surg*. 1981;193:60–66.

Spahn DR, Bouillon B, Cerny V, Duranteau J, Filipescu D, Hunt BJ, Komadina R, Maegele M, Nardi G, Riddez L, Samama CM, Vincent JL, Rossaint R. The European guideline on management of major bleeding and coagulopathy following trauma: fifth edition. *Crit Care*. 2019;23:98. https://ccforum.biomedcentral.com/articles/10.1186/s13054-019-2347-3

Spinelli A, Bonovas S, Burisch J, Kucharzik T, Adamina M, Annese V, Bachmann O, Bettenworth D, Chaparro M, Czuber-Dochan W, Eder P, Ellul P, Fidalgo C, Fiorino G, Gionchetti P, Gisbert JP, Gordon H, Hedin C, Holubar S, Iacucci M, Karmiris K, Katsanos K, Kopylov U, Lakatos PL, Lytras T, Lyutakov I, Noor N, Pellino G, Piovani D, Savarino E, Selvaggi F, Verstockt B, Doherty G, Raine T, Panis Y. ECCO guidelines on therapeutics in ulcerative colitis: surgical treatment. *J Crohns Colitis*. 2022 Feb 23;16(2):179–189. doi: 10.1093/ecco-jcc/jjab177.

Still S, Mencio M, Ontiveros E, Burdick J, Leeds SG. Primary and rescue endoluminal vacuum therapy in the management of esophageal perforations and leaks. *Ann Thorac Cardiovasc Surg*. 2018 Aug 20;24(4):173–179.

Sverdén E, Agréus L, Dunn JM, Lagergren J. Peptic ulcer disease. *BMJ*. 2019 Oct 2;367:l5495. doi: 10.1136/bmj.l5495.

Thornell A, Angenete E, Gonzales E, Heath J, Jess P, Läckberg Z, Ovesen H, Rosenberg J, Skullman S, Haglind E; Scandinavian Surgical Outcomes Research Group, SSORG. Treatment of acute diverticulitis laparoscopic lavage vs. resection (DILALA): study protocol for a randomised controlled trial. *Trials*. 2011 Aug 1;12:186. doi: 10.1186/1745-6215-12-186.

Tripathi D, Stanley AJ, Hayes PC, et al. UK guidelines on the management of variceal haemorrhage in cirrhotic patients. *Gut*. 2015:1–25. doi: 10.1136/gutjnl-2015-309262.

Truelove SC, Witts LJ. Cortisone in ulcerative colitis; final report on a therapeutic trial. *Br Med J*. 1955 Oct 29;2(4947):1041–1048. doi: 10.1136/bmj.2.4947.1041.

5 Endocrine Surgery

Paul C. Dent and Simon Chang-Hao Tsao

Q1. A 29-year-old female presents in the clinic with a history of renal stones and constipation. Her adjusted calcium is 2.79 mmol/L (2.20–2.60 mmol/L). The PTH is 4.7 pmol/L (1.6–6.9 pmol/L), and the vitamin D level is 68 nmol/L (50–120 nmol/L). What is the next most appropriate test?

A. US Renal tract
B. Sestamibi
C. Genetics
D. Urinary metanephrines
E. 24-hour urinary calcium creatinine clearance ratio

Q2. A 52-year-old female presents to your clinic with a slight swelling in the anterior triangle of her neck. There are no swallowing or breathing issues, and her voice has not changed. She has recently had a change in bowel habits and has been investigated for bowel pathology. CEA was 45, though staging CT and colonoscopy were normal. What is the most likely diagnosis?

A. Papillary thyroid cancer
B. Follicular thyroid cancer
C. Medullary thyroid cancer
D. Lymphoma of the thyroid
E. Anaplastic thyroid cancer

Q3. A 43-year-old male taking four antihypertensives having some muscle weakness has been referred to your clinic for review. His serum potassium is 3.2 mmol/L. What is the most appropriate test?

A. Overnight dexamethasone suppression test
B. Aldosterone–renin ratio
C. DHEAS
D. Urinary metanephrines
E. Plasma metanephrines

Q4. A 53-year-old male who has previously had a laparoscopic right hemicolectomy for adenocarcinoma. A follow-up CT shows a new 2 cm mass in the left adrenal gland. The patient does not take any antihypertensives. What is the most appropriate investigation?

A. 24-hour blood pressure monitoring
B. MRI scan with in/out phase protocol
C. PET CT
D. Fine-needle aspiration
E. Overnight dexamethasone test

DOI: 10.1201/9781003221234-5

Q5. A 26-year-old female presents to the endocrine surgical clinic following a referral from the endocrinology team with a TSH that is less than 0.02, a T4 of 49 pmol/L and a T3 of 23 pmol/L. TSH autoantibodies are significantly elevated. The endocrinology team have started her on 200 mg of propylthiouracil daily. This patient is keen to start a family within the next 3 to 6 months. What would be the most appropriate management?
   A.   Carbimazole treatment 40 mg daily
   B.   Continue management propylthiouracil
   C.   Referral for radioactive iodine treatment
   D.   Total thyroidectomy with Lugol's iodine for 1 week prior to surgery
   E.   Stop propylthiouracil before her pregnancy.

Q6. A 48-year-old male has been identified with medullary thyroid cancer measuring 8 mm in the left thyroid lobe following ultrasound and fine-needle aspiration. There are no suspicious lymph nodes within the central or lateral neck. What would be the most appropriate management?
   A.   Left thyroid lobectomy
   B.   Left thyroid lobectomy with central neck dissection
   C.   Total thyroidectomy
   D.   Total thyroidectomy and central neck dissection
   E.   Right thyroid lobectomy with central neck dissection

Q7. A 63-year-old male has been referred to your clinic from the colorectal team following a staging FDG PET scan for his colorectal cancer. This has demonstrated a positive PET hotspot within the right thyroid lobe. What would be the most appropriate management?
   A.   Total thyroidectomy with central neck dissection
   B.   Ultrasound and core biopsy
   C.   Right thyroid lobectomy and selective levels 2–4 lateral neck dissection
   D.   Ultrasound and fine-needle aspiration cytology
   E.   Staging MRI of the neck with chest X-ray

Q8. A 52-year-old female with bilateral adrenal nodular hyperplasia has been referred to your clinic by the endocrinology team with poorly controlled diabetes. The aldosterone/renin ratio is normal, urinary metanephrines are normal and DHEAS is normal. The 9 AM cortisol is 900 nmol/L, and an overnight dexamethasone suppression test value is 268 nmol/L. What would be the most appropriate management?
   A.   Repeat overnight dexamethasone suppression test with CRH suppression.
   B.   Bilateral retroperitoscopic adrenalectomy.
   C.   Mitotane treatment.
   D.   Return to the endocrinology team for consideration of a GLP–1 agonist such as liraglutide.
   E.   MRI adrenal protocol.

Q9. A 39-year-old man is referred to your endocrine surgical clinic with a PTH of 97 pmol/L, an adjusted calcium of 2.99 mmol/L and a vitamin D of 75 nmol/L. His ultrasound demonstrates a left-sided parathyroid adenoma lying posteriorly to the thyroid lobe, and this is co-localised with a sestamibi scan. He is taken to theatre where a left-sided exploration is performed, and during surgery, the superior parathyroid is difficult to dissect free from the thyroid lobe. What would be the most appropriate management?
   A. Left thyroid lobectomy with superior parathyroidectomy
   B. Left thyroid lobectomy with superior and inferior parathyroidectomies
   C. Total thyroidectomy with left superior parathyroidectomy
   D. Bilateral neck exploration with the excision of left superior parathyroid and any other parathyroids appearing abnormal
   E. Left thyroid lobectomy with superior and inferior parathyroidectomies, cervical thymectomy and left level 6 lymphadenectomy

Q10. A 73-year-old female is referred to your endocrine surgical clinic with a biochemical diagnosis of primary hyperparathyroidism and images of localised left parathyroid adenoma. On ultrasound scan, there is a right thyroid nodule which is also sestamibi-positive. Fine-needle aspiration cytology suggests that this right thyroid nodule is THY5, papillary thyroid carcinoma. The patient explains she does not wish to take thyroxine if possible. What would be the most appropriate management?
   A. Right thyroid lobectomy with concurrent left parathyroidectomy
   B. Total thyroidectomy
   C. Left thyroid lobectomy with concurrent left parathyroidectomy
   D. Right thyroid lobectomy with staged left parathyroidectomy
   E. Bilateral neck exploration and parathyroidectomy

Q11. A 59-year-old female referred to you with a 3 cm right thyroid nodule; fine-needle aspirate is Thy 3f. One enlarged right level 3 node showed normally appearing thyroid cells.
      What is the next best management?
   A. CT of the neck
   B. Total thyroidectomy with right selective lateral neck dissection and bilateral central neck dissection
   C. Right hemithyroidectomy with excision biopsy of the right level 3 node
   D. Right hemithyroidectomy only and adjuvant radioactive iodine
   E. CT of the chest, abdomen and pelvis.

Q12. A GP referred a 25-year-old female with hyperthyroidism. She has a resting heart rate of 125; she is anxious and agitated. Ultrasound showed a diffuse vascular thyroid gland without any nodules. What is the next best management?
   A. Urgent subtotal thyroidectomy
   B. Urgent total thyroidectomy
   C. Total thyroidectomy following 1 week of Lugol's
   D. Referral to an endocrinologist for medical management
   E. Referral for urgent radioactive iodine.

Q13. A 33-year-old man presented to his GP with lethargy and nonspecific abdominal pain. He has a palpable left neck nodule. Blood tests showed a corrected calcium of 3.2 mmol/L and a PTH of 67 (2–10). Sestamibi showed an avid left neck nodule around the inferior pole of the thyroid gland. Ultrasound showed a 1.5 cm heterogeneous nodule. The radiologist reported that they cannot distinguish whether it is a thyroid nodule or a parathyroid gland. There is no lateral neck disease. What is the most appropriate management?
   A.   Ultrasound-guided FNA
   B.   Perform a targeted parathyroidectomy
   C.   Left hemithyroidectomy and parathyroidectomy
   D.   Staging PET CT
   E.   Total thyroidectomy with four-gland exploration ± subtotal parathyroidectomy

Q14. A 61-year-old male who had a renal transplant was referred by a renal physician for hypercalcaemia. The renal physician performed initial investigations and showed that the patient's PTH is 12 pmol/L (1.5–6.9 pmol/L), with a corrected calcium of 2.8 mmol/L (2.2–2.6 mmol/L). Sestamibi and ultrasound showed a right-sided parathyroid adenoma. The patient does not have any symptoms of hypercalcaemia. What is the most appropriate management?
   A.   Continue to observe with annual neck ultrasound. Consider an operation when there is more than one abnormal gland.
   B.   Perform a targeted parathyroidectomy.
   C.   Perform a four-gland exploration and subtotal parathyroidectomy.
   D.   Perform a right-sided parathyroid exploration and parathyroidectomy.
   E.   Discharge back to the renal physician and asked to refer back when calcium is above 3.0.

Q15. You performed a diagnostic right thyroid lobectomy on a 45-year-old female for a 2.5 cm Thy3f nodule. Formal histology showed it is follicular thyroid cancer. Preoperative ultrasound did not show any abnormal lateral neck nodes. What is the most appropriate management?
   A.   Consent for completion of thyroidectomy only
   B.   Consent for completion of thyroidectomy with bilateral central neck dissection
   C.   Consent for completion of thyroidectomy, bilateral central neck dissection and right selective neck dissection
   D.   Request TFT, thyroglobulin and thyroglobulin antibodies now
   E.   Discuss the chances of contralateral disease and refer to a radiation oncologist for radioactive iodine.

Q16. A 66-year-old man with hypertension and hypokalaemia presented. The blood test showed a high aldosterone-to-renin ratio. CT scan showed a 1.3 cm nodule in the left adrenal gland, and the HU was 34. What is the most appropriate management?
   A.   Check for PTH level before considering surgery
   B.   Perform a laparoscopic left adrenalectomy
   C.   Check for plasma DHEA and testosterone level
   D.   Request MRI of the adrenal gland
   E.   Request an adrenal-venous sampling.

Q17. A 43-year-old female with long-term, poorly controlled, diabetes, hypertension and Grave's disease was referred to you by her endocrinologist. She has failed medical management for her thyrotoxicosis. You performed a straightforward total thyroidectomy, and all four parathyroid glands were preserved and viable by the end of the operation. However, the next day, this patient developed tetany and cramps. What is the most likely cause of her symptoms?

A. Severe hypothyroidism
B. Hungry bone syndrome
C. Hypoparathyroidism
D. Hyperparathyroidism
E. Refractive thyroid storm

Q18. A 65-year-old man with primary hyperparathyroidism received a focused parathyroidectomy following congruent sestamibi and ultrasound to a left inferior parathyroid adenoma. Histology confirmed parathyroid adenoma. Postoperative PTH and calcium normalised for 5 weeks but returned to the preoperative level. What is the best next approach?

A. Early take back for four-gland explorations within the next 4 weeks.
B. Repeat neck ultrasound then plan surgery 6 months later.
C. 4D-CT then plan surgery 6 months later.
D. Repeat neck ultrasound then early four-gland exploration within the next 4 weeks.
E. Repeat sestamibi and ultrasound and then focused parathyroidectomy if another adenoma is localised, within the next 4 weeks.

Q19. A 54-year-old female who is otherwise fit and healthy was referred to you with multi-nodular goitre. The ultrasound showed multiple U2 nodules in both lobes of the thyroid with a predominant goitre on the right side. A CT scan also showed that the left lobe is only mildly enlarged, but the right lobe reaches down to the level of the aortic arch. She has no symptoms of compression. What would you recommend?

A. Right thyroid lobectomy with potential sternotomy
B. Total thyroidectomy with sternotomy
C. Start on levothyroxine
D. Refer for radioactive iodine
E. External beam radiotherapy

Q20. An 18-year-old boy with an infected cyst in the midline of his neck. You noticed that this cyst moves with tongue movement. What is the most appropriate surgical management for this lesion?

A. Localised cystectomy.
B. Localised cyst marsupialisation.
C. Remove the cyst, its tracts and the thyroid isthmus.
D. Remove the cyst with a fraction of the hyoid bone and track it up towards the tongue.
E. Remove the cyst with total thyroidectomy and its tracks.

ANSWERS

Q1. Option E – 24-hour urinary calcium creatinine clearance ratio.

The serum tests would suggest primary hyperparathyroidism. It would be appropriate to perform a 24-hour urinary collection to confirm that this is not FHH. Once this is completed as this patient is under 30, genetics should be sent to assess for MEN1 as this will affect surgical options. A sestamibi scan should be requested once urinary tests confirm that this is primary hyperparathyroidism. Renal US is performed alongside bone Densitometry as per the current NICE guidelines to review for renal stones (known in this case) and assess cortical bone density.

Q2. Option C – Medullary thyroid cancer.

CEA, together with calcitonin, is a tumour marker associated with medullary thyroid carcinoma. Papillary thyroid carcinoma and follicular thyroid carcinoma are differentiated thyroid cancers and thyroglobulin is the tumour marker used.

Q3. Option B – Aldosterone–renin ratio.

This patient has poorly controlled hypertension and low potassium which is almost certainly related to Conn's syndrome. All of these will need to be done in one form or another, but the aldosterone–renin ratio will be diagnostic. However, the patient will need to only take doxazocin as most other antihypertensives can make assessment difficult.

Q4. Option C – PET CT.

Given the previous history of malignancy, this makes the metastatic disease the most likely differential and a PET CT would be sensible. Fine-needle aspiration should not be performed until a phaeochromocytoma is ruled out using metanephrines.

Q5. Option D – Total thyroidectomy with Lugol's iodine for 1 week prior to surgery.

This patient has been referred for Graves' disease and given that she is keen to start a family within the next 3–6 months the most appropriate management would be a total thyroidectomy with Lugol's iodine treatment for a week prior to surgery. Carbimazole should not be used during pregnancy for its risk of teratogenic effects, and radioactive iodine should not be given to men or women who planned to start a family within the next 6–12 months.

Q6. Option D – Total thyroidectomy and central neck dissection.

The current recommendations for medullary thyroid cancer greater than 5 mm would be a total thyroidectomy and central neck dissection. Lateral neck dissection should be considered if there is cytologically proven metastasis or if calcitonin levels are significantly elevated prior to surgery; however, a DOTATATE PET scan may be advised for staging.

Q7. Option D – Ultrasound and fine-needle aspiration cytology.

FDG avid hotspots within the thyroid have a malignancy risk of 25% and so ultrasound-guided aspiration cytology would be recommended prior to further surgical management.

Q8. Option B – Bilateral retroperitoscopic adrenalectomy.

This patient has poorly controlled diabetes due to excessive cortisol secretion as a result of her bilateral adrenal nodular hyperplasia. Her functional studies show that while the majority are normal her overnight dexamethasone suppression test is not adequate (less than 50 nmol/L), so bilateral retroperitoscopic adrenalectomy is the most appropriate management for this patient.

Q9. Option E – Left thyroid lobectomy with superior and inferior parathyroidectomies, cervical thymectomy and left level 6 lymphadenectomy.

This gentleman has significantly high PTH and adjusted calcium. While his imaging has been concordantly suggesting a left superior parathyroid at surgery. there is a concern that this may be a malignant parathyroid. The recommendation would be a left thyroid lobectomy with *en bloc* excision of the superior and inferior parathyroids, the cervical sinus and left level 6 lymph nodes.

Q10. Option D – Right thyroid lobectomy with staged left parathyroidectomy.

This patient has a right-sided thyroid malignancy which can be found as a positive sestamibi nodule. As she has already had cytology demonstrating this to be malignant, the recommendation would be for her to have a right thyroid lobectomy with a staged left parathyroidectomy at a second operation. This would allow histological examination of the right thyroid lobe as completion of left thyroid lobectomy may be required dependent on the findings. This will take into account her wishes that she does not wish to take thyroxine if at all possible. We would not recommend exploration of the left neck at the same time as the right-sided surgery due to the risk that should a completion thyroidectomy be required this would increase the risk of complications by operating where a previous neck dissection has been performed.

Q11. Option A – CT neck.

This patient has lateral neck disease. It is important to assess the extent of the disease by performing a CT neck. This will determine the extent of the selective neck dissection. If there is no other disease, an appropriate surgical option will be to perform a total thyroidectomy, bilateral central neck dissection and right selective neck dissection (levels II–IV).

Q12. Option D – Referral to an endocrinologist for medical management.

This patient needs to have thyroid toxicity controlled first; she is at risk of thyroid storm if going ahead with immediate surgery. The cause of thyroid toxicity needs to be investigated. Graves' or acute thyroiditis cannot be distinguished by ultrasound alone. Thyroiditis usually can be managed medically.

Q13. Option D – Staging PET CT.

Clinically, this patient has high suspicion of parathyroid carcinoma, which has a high likelihood of metastasis. Metastatic parathyroid carcinoma usually requires medical management of hypercalcaemia rather than surgery as the prognosis is poor.

Q14. Option C – Perform a four-gland exploration and subtotal parathyroidectomy.
       This patient has tertiary hyperparathyroidism, and therefore, it is common to
       have more than one gland disease. It is imperative to explore all four glands and
       remove all the abnormal glands. Put a prolene stitch on the remaining glands. It
       is possible to observe this patient; however, the patient is young and prolonged
       hyperparathyroidism has detrimental effects on bone density in the long term.

Q15. Option A – Consent for completion of thyroidectomy only.
       Follicular thyroid cancer spreads haematogenously; therefore, prophylactic
       neck dissection is not warranted. In order to detect future metastatic disease and
       recurrence, completion of thyroidectomy is required in order for thyroglobulin
       and thyroglobulin antibodies to be reliable. Depending on the further completion
       of histology, she may be referred for consideration of radioactive iodine.

Q16. Option E – Request an adrenal-venous sampling.
       Both adrenal adenoma and adrenal hyperplasia may cause hyperaldosteronism.
       It is vitally important to confirm the pathological gland prior to surgery.

Q17. Option B – Hungry bone syndrome.
       Patients with chronic thyrotoxicosis are in a state of high bone turnover. They
       are at risk of severe hypocalcaemia post-thyroidectomy when bone formation
       exceeds bone resorption.

Q18. Option C – 4D-CT then plan surgery 6 months later.
       Taking back to the theatre more than 2–3 weeks post-initial surgery is
       associated with high morbidity and failed exploration rate. 4D-CT is more
       sensitive than ultrasound ± sestamibi, especially for the extra-thyroidal
       parathyroid gland. To avoid a potential third surgery, most centres will perform
       a four-gland exploration ± removal of the thymus and extra-thyroidal parathyroid
       adenoma if there is any during the second surgery, usually 6 months later.

Q19. Option A – Right thyroid lobectomy with potential sternotomy.
       There are a number of indications for thyroidectomy. These include cosmesis,
       malignancy, toxic nodularity, compression symptoms and retrosternal goitre
       where we are unable to assess whether this is malignant due to the inability of
       performing either an ultrasound scan or FNA of this section. In this situation, it
       would be advisable to discuss with the patient that as this is retrosternal and to the
       level of the arch of the aorta, a right thyroid lobectomy with potential sternotomy
       is indicated. Given her youthful age, a lobectomy will potentially mean 80% of
       patients would not necessarily require levothyroxine post-operatively and will
       also reduce the risks of hypocalcaemia due to hypoparathyroidism.

Q20. Option D – Remove the cyst with a fraction of the hyoid bone and track it up
       towards the tongue. This is a thyroglossal duct cyst. The correct procedure is a
       Sistrunk's.

6 Hepato-Pancreatico-Biliary Surgery

Ajay Belgaumkar, Irena Stefanova,
Nabeel Merali, and Muhammad Fahim

Q1. A 31-year-old woman who is 29 weeks pregnant presents to the emergency department with right upper quadrant pain, fever and jaundice. Her pulse rate is 115, her temperature is 38.9 and blood pressure is 75/40. Her laboratory studies show WCC: 19.1, HB: 105, CRP: 210, Bilirubin: 125, ALP: 690, and ALT: 230. Her USS abdomen demonstrates gallstones within a thin-walled gallbladder and extra and intrahepatic biliary duct dilatation. What is the most appropriate management?
A. Laparoscopic cholecystectomy and CBD exploration
B. Conservative management with antibiotics and intravenous fluids only
C. Open cholecystectomy
D. Urgent MRCP followed by ERCP ± sphincterotomy ± stent
E. MRCP and laparoscopic cholecystectomy post delivery

Q2. A 54-year-old man presents with 2 days history of right upper quadrant pain, vomiting and fever. His laboratory studies show WCC: 16.7, CRP: 170, bilirubin: 35, ALP: 230 and ALT: 150. His USS shows a thickened-wall gallbladder containing gallstones and pericholecystic fluid, with no intra- or extrahepatic biliary duct dilatation. The patient is admitted and commenced on intravenous antibiotics. His liver function tests the following day are bilirubin: 23, ALP: 190 and ALT: 90. What is the most appropriate management?
A. Laparoscopic cholecystectomy and on-table cholangiogram on this admission
B. Laparoscopic cholecystectomy only
C. Open cholecystectomy
D. Urgent ERCP
E. MRCP followed by ERCP

Q3. A 69-year-old woman presents to the emergency department with right upper quadrant pain, fever and jaundice. Her LFTs are bilirubin: 140, ALP: 790 and ALT 300. Her USS shows acute cholecystitis with normal-size CBD but significant intrahepatic biliary duct dilatation. MRCP demonstrates Mirizzi type 2. What is the appropriate management?
A. MRCP and ERCP are sufficient to manage Mirizzi type 2
B. Urgent ERCP ± stent followed by laparoscopic/open subtotal cholecystectomy ± closure of cholecystocholedochal fistula
C. Laparoscopic cholecystectomy during the same hospital admission
D. Conservative management with antibiotics only
E. PTC only

DOI: 10.1201/9781003221234-6

Q4. A 69-year-old male patient presents to the upper GI clinic with 3 months history of abdominal pain, back pain and anorexia. A TWR CT CAP scan shows likely IPMN in the pancreatic body. What are the next steps of diagnosis/management?

A. Discharge from UGI clinic without a follow-up as IPMN are benign pancreatic lesions
B. Book for pancreatic resection at the earliest opportunity
C. Request tumour markers (CEA, CA 19-9), MRCP and EUS+ FNA to assess for high-risk criteria
D. Request an MRI pancreas
E. Repeat CT in 6 months

Q5. A 19-year-old male presents as a trauma call following a motorcycle accident and blunt trauma to the abdomen. He undergoes ATLS protocol assessment and immediate management and undergoes CT trauma series which demonstrates grade III pancreatic injury. Which statement describes best the most appropriate management?

A. Admit for close observation and serum amylase
B. Emergency laparotomy and pancreaticoduodenectomy
C. Exploratory laparotomy, primary suture of pancreatic laceration and drain insertion
D. Emergency laparotomy, distal pancreatectomy and splenectomy
E. Emergency ERCP

Q6. A 63-year-old woman with a background of breast cancer and a previous mastectomy followed by adjuvant chemotherapy is referred to the upper GI clinic with right upper quadrant pain and suspected gallstone disease. She undergoes an ultrasound abdomen which demonstrates three hypoechoic ill-defined lesions in liver segments 4 and 5. CT of the chest, abdomen and pelvis confirms liver lesions and shows no other abnormalities. What is the most appropriate management?

A. Organise follow-up USS in 6 months
B. Refer for consideration of liver resection
C. Refer to oncology for chemotherapy
D. Organise liver biopsy and add to HPB MDT
E. Discharge from the clinic without follow-up

Q7. A 41-year-old female patient who has been using oral contraception for the last 7 years has an incidental finding on a CT scan of the focal liver lesion with a central scar suspicious of FNH. She is asymptomatic. MRI of the liver is inconclusive in differentiating between focal nodular hyperplasia (FNH) and hepatocellular adenoma (HCA). Which of the following statements regarding this patient's management is least likely to be correct?

A. Liver biopsy is required to differentiate FNH from HCA
B. Liver biopsy is not indicated as both FNH and HCA are benign liver lesions
C. In individuals with FNH the ongoing use of contraceptives is not contraindicated
D. Individuals with asymptomatic and stable FNH who are not on oral contraception do not require follow-up
E. Symptomatic FNH can be treated by partial hepatic resection, embolisation or radiofrequency ablation

Q8. A 55-year-old male patient presents in the clinic with abdominal discomfort, nausea and early satiety. USS shows a complex hepatic cyst. CT and MRI confirm heterogeneous septations, irregular papillary growths and thick walls. What is the most appropriate course of action?
   A. Regular follow-up with annual USS as this is not a solid liver lesion
   B. Interventional radiology-guided aspiration/biopsy to establish histological diagnosis
   C. Complete surgical excision is required
   D. No follow-up required, discharge from the clinic
   E. Laparoscopic/open deroofing is required

Q9. A 64-year-old male patient undergoes an ultrasound which shows a 3 cm and a 4 cm solid focal liver lesion. Further MRI liver demonstrates liver lesions of the same size in seg 4B and seg 3 suspicious of hepatocellular carcinoma. What is the most appropriate treatment option?
   A. There are no curative surgical options as this is multifocal HCC, so this patient should be referred to oncology for sorafenib
   B. Right hemihepatectomy
   C. Left hemihepatectomy
   D. Chemoembolisation with curative intent
   E. Palliation

Q10. A 76-year-old female patient is recently diagnosed with HCC. Their CT and MRI demonstrate a 6 cm lesion in seg 4B and a 4 cm lesion in seg 7 with invasion to the left portal vein. What is the most appropriate management?
   A. Right hemicolectomy
   B. Left hemicolectomy
   C. Palliation
   D. Chemoembolisation with curative intent
   E. There are no curative surgical options as this is multifocal HCC, so this patient should be referred to oncology for sorafenib

Q11. A 50-year-old gentleman presented today only 2 days following elective day-case laparoscopic cholecystectomy with symptoms of worsening abdominal pain and fever. On examination, he is found how to have hypotension and tachycardia with tenderness and guarding throughout his abdomen. What would be the most appropriate management plan?
   A. Urgent ERCP
   B. MRCP
   C. Ultrasound of abdomen and pelvis
   D. CT scan of abdomen and pelvis with oral contrast
   E. Diagnostic laparoscopy

Q12. A 58-year-old man presents with painless jaundice with an unremarkable past medical history and is otherwise fit and healthy. Her laboratory studies show WC:C 7.2, HB: 105, CRP: 35, bilirubin: 230, ALP: 690, and ALT: 230. CT and MRCP demonstrate a hilar cholangiocarcinoma involving both right and left hepatic ducts up to secondary biliary radicals bilaterally. What is the most appropriate management?

    A. Organise a EUS and biopsy as part of planning curative surgery

    B. Perform a bile duct resection, hepatic resection and portal lymphadenectomy

    C. Perform a pancreaticoduodenectomy

    D. Perform a local bile duct excision and orthotopic liver transplantation (OLT)

    E. Perform a palliative biliary decompression such as a percutaneous or endoscopic biliary stent placement

Q13. You are performing a laparoscopic cholecystectomy. Which of the following statements is false?

    A. Dissection of the hepatocystic triangle, bounded by the gallbladder wall, cystic duct, and common hepatic duct, to obtain the "critical view of safety"

    B. Critical view of safety should be achieved prior to clipping and dividing tubular structures

    C. Avoid dissecting down to the cystic duct-common bile duct junction

    D. Intraoperative cholangiography (IOC) should be accomplished before beginning common bile duct (CBD) exploration

    E. Rouviere's sulcus is a fissure on the liver that corresponds to the level of the porta hepatis and dissection below this level is safe

Q14. A 52-year-old man had an uneventful laparoscopic cholecystectomy for symptomatic gallstone disease. He presents with upper abdominal pain and vomiting on day 5. His laboratory studies show WCC: 17.2, HB: 105, CRP: 335 and bilirubin: 180. His observations are HR: 105, B/P: 120/70 and temperature: 38.9. CT imaging shows a large loculated volume of fluid within the Morrison pouch and gastrohepatic ligament. What is the most appropriate management?

    A. Reconstruction surgery, Roux-en-Y hepaticojejunostomy

    B. Perform an ERCP for biliary drainage

    C. T-tube drainage of the CBD at the site of the injury

    D. CT-guided drainage of intra-abdominal fluid collection and transfer to a tertiary HPB Centre

    E. Percutaneous transhepatic cholangiography to delineate the intrahepatic ducts

Q15. A 48-year-old lady presented with right upper quadrant pain and on examination, a palpable gallbladder was noted. She is an unremarkable past medical history. Her laboratory studies show WCC: 8, HB: 105, CRP<4 and bilirubin: 19. A CT scan revealed a polypoid mass protruding into the gallbladder lumen with diffuse thickening of the gallbladder wall, indicative of gallbladder carcinoma with no evidence of metastasis. What is the most appropriate management?

    A. Organise an MRCP to evaluate the liver parenchyma and bile duct

    B. Perform an ERCP and metal stent

    C. Diagnostic laparoscopy and proceed to extended cholecystectomy with wedge resection of segment 4B/5

    D. Routine laparoscopic cholecystectomy for a T2 tumour

    E. Refer for palliative chemotherapy

Q16. A 42-year-old lady presented with a typical triad of abdominal pain, jaundice, and right upper quadrant mass. She has an unremarkable past medical history. MRI of the pancreas/MRCP revealed a type 1 choledochal cyst characterised by fusiform dilation of the CBD. What is the most appropriate management?
   A. Single-stage complete excision of the cyst, cholecystectomy with hepaticojejunostomy
   B. Perform ERCP/EUS to further characterise the cyst
   C. Low risk of malignancy
   D. Simple cyst excision
   E. Management with ERCP and cyst mucosal biopsy

Q17. A 39-year-old lady had an inpatient endoscopic retrograde cholangiopancrea-tography (ERCP) for obstructive jaundice secondary to choledocholithiasis. Within 24 hours she developed severe epigastric pain with an amylase of 2,800 and was managed for acute pancreatitis. On day 4, CT imaging revealed peripancreatic necrosis with splenic vein thrombosis. What is the most appropriate management?
   A. Start full anticoagulation in view of the splenic vein thrombosis
   B. According to the Atlanta classification, acute pancreatitis can be divided into three categories
   C. Initial management consists of supportive care with fluid resuscitation, pain control, and nutritional support
   D. Total parenteral nutrition (TPN) is the choice of nutrition in moderate to severe pancreatitis
   E. Organise minimal invasive percutaneous drainage of the pancreatic necrosis

Q18. A 75-year-old male presented with complicated necrotising pancreatitis, with a 4-week history of worsening epigastric pain and vomiting. His laboratory studies show WCC: 31, HB: 105, CRP: 350 and bilirubin: 32. He developed a large pseudocyst that caused an obstruction of the biliary tract as well as gastric outlet obstruction. This pseudocyst became infected, as evidenced by extensive gas within the cyst on CT imaging and is now pyrexic. What is the most appropriate management?
   A. Perform open necrosectomy
   B. Endoscopic cyst gastrostomy, fully covered and self-expandable metal stent
   C. Continue with conservative management with antibiotics and enteral nutrition
   D. Perform fine needle aspiration of the necrotic collection
   E. Perform an ERCP and plastic stent

Q19. A 47-year-old lady presented with severe painless obstructive jaundice and on CT imaging is found to have pancreatic ductal adenocarcinoma at the head of the pancreas. Staging investigations are negative for metastatic disease. Her laboratory studies show WCC: 15, HB: 105, CRP: 150, bilirubin: 390 and CA19-9 256. What is the most appropriate management?
   A. ERCP and metal-covered stent
   B. ERCP alone
   C. PTC alone
   D. Perform pylorus-preserving pancreaticoduodenectomy (PPPD)
   E. Refer for neoadjuvant chemotherapy

Q20. A 52-year-old gentleman presents with a 3-month history of unintentional weight loss and nonspecific abdominal pain. His blood tests are unremarkable, other than a raised CA19-9 of 58. CT imaging confirms a locally advanced pancreatic head mass with solid tumour contact with a SMA ≤180 degrees. EUS and FNA biopsy confirms PDAC. What is the most appropriate management?

A. Exploratory laparotomy and PPPD
B. Deemed unresectable
C. Refer for neoadjuvant chemotherapy
D. Perform ERCP
E. Perform staging laparoscopy

Q21. A 52-year-old man presented with impending large bowel obstruction secondary to low rectal cancer. CT imaging revealed a large segment VII lesion consisting net with colorectal liver metastasis. Confirmed on MRI of the liver, it appears to be solitary. What is the most appropriate management?

A. Colorectal first approach
B. Simultaneous resection
C. Liver-first approaches
D. Two-staged approach
E. Refer for neoadjuvant therapy

Q22. A 53-year-old woman with performance status 0 and a recent diagnosis of metastatic pancreatic cancer, presents to the emergency department with multiple episodes of vomiting. CT scan of the abdomen and pelvis reveals gastric outlet obstruction at the level of D3 caused by the progression of pancreatic tumour, with liver metastasis. What would be the next step in the management of this patient?

A. Gastrojejunostomy
B. Duodenal Stenting
C. Whipple's procedure
D. Referral to oncology for chemotherapy
E. Referral to palliative care team

Q23. While performing a difficult cholecystectomy for acute cholecystitis, you have encountered torrential bleeding. Which of the following is likely to be injured?

A. Cystic artery
B. Left hepatic artery
C. Right hepatic artery
D. Hepatic artery proper
E. Portal vein

Q24. A 22-year-old woman with a known history of recurrent biliary colic and a BMI of 35 kg/m² is admitted with right upper quadrant pain, fever and localised tenderness in the right hypochondrium. The blood test report shows bilirubin: 63, ALP: 208, ALT: 173, CRP: 53 and WCC: 1D. She has been started on co-amoxiclav (according to the Trust protocol) and kept nil by mouth. What is the ideal next step in this patient's management?

A. Emergency laparoscopic cholecystectomy with on-table cholangiogram
B. Ultrasound of the abdomen
C. ERCP
D. MRCP
E. CT with intravenous contrast

Q25. During the investigation for suspected left-sided renal colic, a 47-year-old fit and healthy woman of Chinese origin has an abdominal ultrasound. This shows three gallbladder polyps with a maximum size of 5mm in a thin-walled gallbladder and normal biliary tree. She has never had any typical biliary symptoms and has no history or family history of gastrointestinal problems. How would you manage this patient?

A. Offer cholecystectomy due to ethnicity
B. Discharge with reassurance
C. MRCP
D. CT with intravenous contrast
E. Repeat ultrasound scan in 12 months

Q26. A fit and healthy 67-year-old woman undergoes routine day-case laparoscopic cholecystectomy for biliary colic. Two weeks after surgery, the histology shows that there is an incidental gallbladder cancer at the posterior (liver side) wall. The report describes the tumour as T2. How do you manage this patient?

A. Inform patient of histology results, reassure and discharge
B. Refer to a clinical oncologist for targeted radiotherapy to the gallbladder bed
C. Refer to hepatobiliary surgeon for consideration of liver resection – wedge resection or formal Sg IVb/V resection
D. Refer to a medical oncologist for adjuvant chemotherapy with folfirinox
E. Inform patient of histology results and arrange staging CT in 3 months

Q27. A 58-year-old, fit and healthy man presents a 3-week history of malaise with painless obstructive jaundice. Blood tests include bilirubin: 145, WCC: 9, CRP: 15, ALP: 350, ALT: 180, and Hb: 120. Staging CT shows a 2cm mass in the head of the pancreas with gross dilatation of the biliary tree and pancreatic ducts. The portal vein and superior mesenteric artery are unremarkable and no metastases are identified. How would you proceed next?

A. ERCP with an uncovered metal stent, referral to oncology
B. PET scan followed by pancreaticoduodenectomy
C. Pancreaticoduodenectomy
D. Endoscopic ultrasound and biopsy
E. PET scan, endoscopic ultrasound and diagnostic laparoscopy

Q28. A 68-year-old woman, with performance status 0, presents with a new B.5cm peripheral liver lesion in segment 6 on surveillance CT CAP, 2 years following laparoscopic anterior resection of T2N1M0 rectal cancer. CT PET shows that the lesion is FDG avid and has no other sites of disease. How would you proceed?

A. Liver biopsy to confirm the diagnosis
B. Referral to oncology for palliative chemotherapy
C. Referral to oncology for neoadjuvant chemotherapy before consideration of resection
D. Right hemihepatectomy
E. Laparoscopic non-anatomical segment 6 resection

Q29. Following ERCP to retrieve a CBD stone, a 47-year-old woman presents 12 hours later to the emergency department with signs of hypotension, rebound tenderness and guarding throughout the abdomen. CT of the abdomen shows a significant volume of free air and fluid around the liver. ERCP report states "Unable to access papilla, so needle-knife sphincterotomy performed. Unable to get a clear picture of bile duct stones, so plastic stent deployed. For repeat ERCP in 1 week." What is the next step?

   A. Repeat ERCP

   B. Keep nil by mouth, IV antibiotics and fluids and arrange radiology drainage asap

   C. Emergency exploratory laparotomy + proceed

   D. Diagnostic laparoscopy and washout

   E. Transfer to hepatobiliary centre

Q30. Which of the following is not a part of the Child-Pugh classification of perioperative risks in liver surgery?

   A. Bilirubin

   B. Ascites

   C. Creatinine

   D. Encephalopathy

   E. INR

Q31. While performing a laparoscopic cholecystectomy, which one of the following structures is at the highest risk of injury?

   A. CBD

   B. Hepatic artery

   C. Portal vein

   D. Right hepatic duct

   E. Left gastric artery

Q32. In relation to variations in the origin of the hepatic artery, the right hepatic artery arises from

   A. Splenic artery

   B. Gastroduodenal artery

   C. Superior mesenteric artery

   D. Coeliac trunk

   E. Left gastric artery

Q33. While performing a laparotomy for blunt abdominal trauma in a 28-year-old man, there is profuse bleeding from the hepatic veins. Which of the following hepatic veins can be exposed fully?

   A. Right hepatic vein

   B. Left hepatic vein

   C. Inferior hepatic vein

   D. Middle hepatic vein

   E. None of the hepatic veins can be exposed

Q34. A 47-year-old man undergoes pancreaticoduodenectomy for adenocarcinoma of the pancreas. Which of the following is not a risk factor for the development of pancreatic fistula?
A. Large pancreatic duct diameter
B. Renal comorbidity
C. Multi-visceral resection
D. Prolonged operative time
E. High BMI

Q35. A 58-year-old man has recently been diagnosed with carcinoma of the head of the pancreas. Which of the following will be an indication of pre-operative biliary drainage?
A. To reduce peri-operative mortality
B. To improve median survival
C. To institute neoadjuvant therapy
D. To reduce hospital length of stay
E. None of the above

Q36. A 35-year-old lady underwent an ultrasound scan of her abdomen for upper abdominal pain. She is found to have a well-defined vascular lesion in the right lobe of the liver. Which of the following will be the most useful investigation to reach a diagnosis?
A. CT scan of the abdomen
B. Alpha fetoprotein and liver function tests
C. US-guided biopsy
D. MRI of liver
E. Technetium-99m colloid scan

Q37. Regarding pancreatic tumours, which one of the following has the least potential for malignant transformation?
A. Solid papillary neoplasm
B. Serous cystadenoma
C. Mucinous cystic neoplasm
D. Intraductal papillary mucinous neoplasm
E. Pancreaticoblastoma

Q38. A 65-year-old man is admitted to the ITU following a diagnosis of severe acute pancreatitis. Which of the following will not improve the mortality rate in cases of severe acute pancreatitis?
A. Aggressive IV fluid replacement
B. Enteral nutritional support
C. Use of prophylactic antibiotics
D. Intensive organ support
E. Intervention for pancreatic necrosis

Q39. A 43-year-old male has presented to the A&E with symptoms and signs suggestive of obstructive jaundice. He has a history of elective cholecystectomy for gallstone disease. Which one of the following is the least likely cause of his obstructive jaundice?

A. Ascending cholangitis
B. Thermal injury from the use of elector diathermy during the procedure
C. Ligation of left hepatic duct
D. Ligation of right hepatic duct
E. Retained/recurrence of stones in CBD

Q40. A 62-year-old lady underwent an *en bloc* resection of the spleen for a malignant tumour of the splenic flexure of the colon. Which of the following abnormal findings on peripheral blood film will not be seen?

A. Howell-Jolly bodies
B. Target cells
C. Ecchinocytes
D. Bite cells
E. Pappenheimer bodies

Q41. A 35-year-old of age man was involved in a road traffic accident and had sustained blunt trauma to the abdomen. He underwent laparotomy and splenectomy for grade 4 splenic injury. Which of the following is the most common early complication following this procedure?

A. Acute gastric dilatation
B. Pancreatitis
C. Overwhelming post-splenectomy sepsis
D. Thromboembolic event
E. Atelectasis

Q42. A 51-year-old gentleman is admitted with the diagnosis of alcoholic pancreatitis. Two days later, he becomes distressed with a pulse rate of 130 bpm, BP=100/65, T=38°C and RR of 28/minute. ABGs show a pH of 7.19, pO_2=7.9, and pCO_2=5.8. The most likely explanation for his clinical deterioration is:

A. Septic shock
B. Infected pancreatic pseudocyst
C. Acute alcohol withdrawal
D. Pulmonary embolism
E. ARDS

Q43. A 32-year-old woman presents to the A&E with an acute onset of severe upper abdominal pain associated with vomiting. She has recently been started on a high dose of steroids and azathioprine for acute exacerbation of her Crohn's disease. Which one of the following is the most likely cause of her symptoms?

A. Toxic megacolon
B. Perforated peptic ulcer
C. Obstruction of small bowel
D. Acute pancreatitis
E. Acute cholecystitis

Q44. To mobilise the left lobe of the liver which of the following ligaments needs to be divided?
   A. Left triangular ligament
   B. Right triangular ligament
   C. Superior leave of falciform ligament
   D. Posterior leaf of filiform ligament
   E. Greater omentum

Q45. A 62-year-old lady underwent a left hemicolectomy for a malignant tumour of the splenic flexure of the colon. During the procedure, there was an inadvertent injury to the spleen. The operating surgeon plans for splenectomy to control the bleeding. Which one of the following is not true regarding an iatrogenic injury to the spleen?
   A. Improper traction on the spleen against its peritoneal attachments is the most common mechanism of intraoperative injury.
   B. Capsular tears are the most common type of injury.
   C. The upper pole of the spleen is more commonly injured, owing to its orientation and the greater concentration of peritoneal attachments.
   D. Hilar injury is best managed by splenectomy.
   E. Splenic preservation could be considered in all cases.

Q46. A 51-year-old gentleman is admitted with the diagnosis of alcoholic pancreatitis. Two days later, he becomes distressed with a pulse rate of 130bpm, BP = 100/65 mmHg, T = 38°C and RR of 28/minute. ABGs show a pH of 7.19, $pO_2 = 7.9$ and $pCO_2 = E.8$. The indications for pancreatic protocol CT scans will include which one of the following?
   A. For a significant clinical deterioration and elevated CRP
   B. For suspicion of local pancreatic complications
   C. For suspected bowel ischaemia
   D. For abdominal compartment syndrome
   E. All of the above

Q47. A 64-year-old woman is being managed in intensive care settings with the diagnosis of severe acute alcoholic pancreatitis for the last 3–4 weeks. Her CT scan reveals pancreatic necrosis with multiple fluid collections. Which one of the following will be an indication of laparotomy in this case?
   A. For a significant clinical deterioration and elevated CRP
   B. For suspicion of local pancreatic complications
   C. Ongoing large bore drainage and irrigation of pancreatic necrosis
   D. Severe abdominal compartment syndrome
   E. All of the above

Q48. A 54-year-old lady with a known history of long-standing ulcerative colitis is referred with symptoms of feeling generally weak and very unwell. She appears deeply jaundiced with abdominal distension. A CT scan of the chest, abdomen and pelvis confirms caecal/ascending colon tumour with liver metastasis. Which of the following is considered a contraindication to resection of colorectal liver metastasis?

    A.   Multiple diffuse metastases
    B.   Metastases larger than 5cm
    C.   A future liver remnant (FLR) of 25% pre-operative volume
    D.   Unresectable extrahepatic malignancy
    E.   All of the above

ANSWERS

Q1. Option D – Urgent MRCP followed by ERCP ± sphincterotomy ± stent.

Gallstone disease is the most common gastrointestinal disease in developed countries and is present in up to 15%–20% of the population. It is the second most common non-obstetric emergency, affecting up to 12% of pregnant women with a risk of recurrence. Up to 3% of pregnant women require a cholecystectomy in the first year after delivery. Gallstone disease has a high risk of developing associated complications, and maternal mortality can be up to 37% with gallstone pancreatitis.

Endoscopic retrograde cholangiopancreatography and cholecystectomy can be performed safely in the second trimester when the chance of miscarriage is relatively low and the risk of radiation-induced injury to the developing foetus is also probably lower. Although typically conservative management is preferred, laparoscopic cholecystectomy in the second trimester is both safe and technically straightforward. There is no UK guidance, both American and European obstetric guidelines support early cholecystectomy to avoid further complications later in pregnancy. In the third trimester, although general anaesthesia is safe for the mother and foetus, lack of space may make surgery difficult. Early induction of labour followed by cholecystectomy may be considered, especially after 35 weeks of gestation when risks to the foetus are minimal.

Q2. Option A – Laparoscopic cholecystectomy and on-table-cholangiogram on this admission.

Patients with abnormal LFTs but only slightly elevated bilirubin and a non-dilated biliary tract on ultrasound are associated with a low risk of CBD stones, so it is safe to proceed directly to LC. Although some surgeons may prefer to have pre-operative identification of CBD stones (by MRCP or EUS) and duct clearance by ERCP prior to LC, further investigation may introduce an unnecessary delay in management, increased costs, resource utilisation and length of stay. The presence of CBD stones is around 10% in this group of patients and the status of the CBD should where possible be clarified by IOC or laparoscopic ultrasound. Where IOC has not been performed, if LFTs remain abnormal post-operatively, they should be investigated by MRCP or EUS.

If CBD stones are found at surgery, the surgeon has several options. Multiple systematic reviews and meta-analyses show that a single-staged procedure by laparoscopic bile duct exploration is safe and cost-effective. This may not always be possible due to theatre logistics and available expertise. Secure closure of the cystic duct with subsequent postoperative ERCP either during the same admission or within 1–2 weeks post-LC is an alternative approach in non-obstructed biliary ducts. Intraoperative ERCP, antegrade stenting of the CBD (with subsequent postoperative ERCP) and Open BDE are evidence-based alternatives.

Patients with a CBD >10 mm and abnormal LFTs with elevated bilirubin represent those at the highest risk of CBD stones. Pre-operative imaging of CBD with MRCP or EUS will identify CBD stones in ~30%, permitting CBD clearance pre-operatively by ERCP or planned LCBDE. However, the most cost-effective algorithm for treatment in centres with the appropriate skill mix remains to proceed to LC and OTC without pre-op investigation, as the majority of patients will not have CBD stones, and the treatment options for managing CBD stones listed above may still be applied. At present, a large-scale multicentre randomised controlled trial is being conducted looking at the role of MRCP in patients with low to moderate pre-operative risk of CBD stones (undilated CBD, bilirubin <50, ALT and/or ALP <2x ULN; The Sunflower Trial).

There should be a locally agreed patient pathway for managing patients in these various scenarios dependent upon local skills and facilities.

Q3. Option B – Urgent ERCP±stent followed by laparoscopic/open subtotal cholecystectomy±closure of cholecystocholedochal fistula.

Csendes classification:

- Type I: extrinsic compression of the common hepatic duct (CHD)
- Type Ia: by impacted gallstone in the gallbladder neck or cystic duct
- Type Ib: if the cystic duct is absent 7
- Type II: erosion of CHD wall and formation of cholecystocholedochal fistula (up to one-third of CHD wall circumference is involved)
- Type III: up to two-thirds of CHD wall circumference is involved in a cholecystocholedochal fistula
- Type IV: entire CHD wall is involved in a cholecystocholedochal fistula
- Type V: any of the above with cholecysto-enteric fistula

The main diagnostic issue is determining if the CHD is intact and obstruction is caused by extrinsic compression (type 1 or "Classic" Mirizzi) or if there is a common cavity between the gallbladder and CHD. MRCP is very useful in the workup to help determine biliary anatomy but may not always accurately determine the extent of cholecysto-choledochal fistula. ERCP is considered a gold standard diagnostic tool for Mirizzi syndrome with >70% sensitivity. Additionally, ERCP and biliary decompression allows the drainage of biliary sepsis, stent placement and further time for patient optimisation. However, ERCP can also be associated with devastating complications, so it should be reserved for jaundiced and septic patients where risks of proceeding straight to definitive surgical management may not be safe.

Although traditionally, open surgery was considered the technique of choice for the management of Mirizzi syndrome, increasing confidence means that laparoscopy can be safely considered as an initial approach. In type I, total or subtotal cholecystectomy may be performed, without the need for dissection of the main biliary tree. When severe inflammation impedes the safe dissection of the Calot triangle, partial or subtotal cholecystectomy can be performed. Various techniques of subtotal cholecystectomy are described within the Tokyo Guidelines, including fundus-first and middle-first approaches. The remnant gallbladder may be closed ("reconstituting") or left open ("fenestrating"), with a drain left to control any postoperative bile leak.

In some cases, T-tube may be inserted or choledochoplasty in order to maintain the continuity of the bile duct. However, if there is a significant loss of duct integrity (>50% in type III and IV), then Roux-en-Y hepaticojejunostomy is the preferred method of biliary reconstruction. Thus, MRCP, ERCP and CT scan should be considered together to stage the type of Mirizzi syndrome and decide if specialist hepatobiliary expertise may be needed before embarking on surgery.

Q4. Option C – Request tumour markers (CEA, CA 19-9), MRCP and EUS+ FNA to assess for high-risk criteria.

IPMNs are epithelial neoplasms that affect either the main pancreatic duct or one of its branches and produce mucin. Main-duct IPMNs are more likely to exhibit severe dysplasia/invasion than lesions occurring in branches. Family history is a well-established risk factor for the development of these lesions. Some conditions, such as Peutz-Jaegers, are more strongly associated than others.

Although most are incidental findings on cross-sectional imaging for other indications such as renal colic, symptoms of IPMNs include abdominal pain, back pain, anorexia, weight loss and recurrent episodes of pancreatitis.

The risk of malignancy in IPMNs is difficult to accurately determine without invasive investigation. Broadly, main-duct and mixed-type IPMN are associated with rates of 35%–75% malignancy, whereas side-branch IPMN is lower, between 15% and 25%. Along with morphological characteristics such as enhancing mural nodules and the extent of pancreatic duct dilatation, size is an important criterion, with lesions <10 mm unlikely to harbour malignancy potential, and lesions >40 mm diameter more likely to be malignant. Repeated surveillance imaging may be required, although the long-term safety and accuracy of various surveillance regimens have not been determined. European guidelines have recently been published which may help to standardise follow-up.

Q5. Option D – Emergency laparotomy, distal pancreatectomy and splenectomy.

Grading the severity of pancreatic injury: grade I – minor contusion or laceration with no duct injury, grade II – major contusion or laceration with no duct injury, grade III – transection or major laceration with duct disruption in the distal pancreas, grade IV – transection of the proximal pancreas or major laceration with associated injury to the ampulla and grade V – Massive disruption of the pancreatic head.

Grade III injuries generally require distal pancreatectomy and splenectomy with drainage. In children, effort should be made to preserve the spleen, if possible, because of the potential for overwhelming post-splenectomy infection. Given the difficulty in dissecting the pancreatic tail and possible bleeding from tributaries, it is advocated that concurrent splenectomy is performed in adults to minimise operating time in unstable patients. There have been no prospective randomised trials comparing stapling with non-absorbable sutures for closing the body of the pancreas. In cases of a clean grade III transection, the pancreas can be conserved.

A jejunal Roux loop can be anastomosed to the body of the pancreas and the distal part of the head of the pancreas can be sutured closed.

In centres with specific expertise, endoscopic pancreatic duct stenting may be attempted to bridge the disrupted duct, with surgery reserved in the event the distal pancreatic duct cannot be accessed.

Q6. Option B – Refer for consideration of liver resection.

Patients with single-site breast liver metastases may benefit from liver resection. Workup should be directed at establishing there are no other sites of disease, with a bone scan and CT PET, before confirming the patient's cardiorespiratory fitness and suitability for surgery. Multiple case series confirm survival post-liver resection is comparable to surgery for colorectal liver metastases in highly selected patients, although randomised controlled trials have not been performed. The role of pre-operative downstaging/neoadjuvant chemotherapy has not been established but may be considered, depending on the pattern of disease, surgical resectability and timing of progression in relation to previous treatment.

Q7. Option B – Liver biopsy is not indicated as both FNH and HCA are benign liver lesions.

Although 20%–40% of cases of FNH may present with symptoms, most are discovered incidentally. FNH is noted primarily in women in their 40s and 50s and may be associated with oral contraceptive pills, hormone replacement therapy and other medications with oestrogen-stimulating properties such as raloxifene.

Identification of classic FNH by way of its "spoke-wheel" central scar on cross-sectional imaging is relatively straightforward. The main differential diagnosis of concern is a hepatocellular adenoma, which carries a greater risk of rupture and malignant transformation.

The diagnostic accuracy of MRI for FNH has improved because of the improvement in hepatobiliary contrast agents, such as Primovist. Most cases of FNH are asymptomatic and stable over time. Occurrences of HCC and spontaneous rupture are rare, so conservative management is appropriate unless there is another indication, such as symptomatic larger lesions or diagnostic uncertainty. Lesions over 5 cm in diameter and those in males should be considered for resection, as risks of malignancy are higher.

Although liver resection is the most common intervention, embolisation and radiofrequency ablation have more recently been utilised as they are associated with fewer complications and lower morbidity. Follow-up annual US for 2–3 years is prudent in women diagnosed with FNH who wish to continue OCP use. Individuals with a firm diagnosis of FNH who are not using OCP do not require follow-up imaging. Hepatocellular adenomas should be resected in patients who are fit for surgery.

A biopsy is not recommended in patients fit for liver resection, due to the risk of seeding. Although PET scan is increasingly used in patients with a previous history of malignancy, FDG avidity is not typically used in primary incidental liver lesions as a criterion for resection.

Q8. Option C – Complete surgical excision is required.

Although rare, biliary cystadenoma (BC) is the most common form of a primary hepatic cystic neoplasm. BCs are thought to be precursors to the development of biliary cystadenocarcinoma (BCA), although it is difficult to predict progression or clearly identify characteristics that herald such progression. Although symptoms are rare, they are often correlated with the increasing size of the lesions leading to mass effect and abdominal discomfort, nausea, early satiety or anorexia. Smaller BC is typically discovered incidentally on imaging.

US typically shows irregular walls and internal septations forming loculi. US is most sensitive in identifying these internal septations. If a complex cyst is found on US, cross-sectional imaging with CT and MRI should be obtained. CT and MRI can help confirm the findings of heterogeneous septations, irregular papillary growths and thickened cyst walls. The cysts are typically hyper-intense on T2 weighting, although because of mucinous content they may appear heterogeneous.

Aspiration and biopsy are not recommended for focusing the differential because it has limited sensitivity and can disseminate malignancy if there is underlying BCA. Although imaging can suggest the possibility of BC or BCA, surgical resection is ultimately necessary to confirm and treat the suspected BC or BCA.

Q9. Option C – Left hemihepatectomy.

There are multiple therapeutic modalities for HCC, which include surgical options [resection or liver transplantation (LT)], and ablative electrochemical therapies (e.g., radiofrequency ablation or ethanol injection). Non-ablative treatment includes catheter-based embolic therapies (e.g., chemoembolisation and radioembolisation) and non-catheter-based therapy such as stereotactic body radiotherapy (SBRT). Finally, systemic therapy in the current era comprises solely of sorafenib, a multikinase inhibitor, and is non-curative. These therapeutic modalities can be broadly classified by the therapeutic intent of attempting to cure or control the tumour.

Surgical and ablative therapies are performed with curative intent, while the majority of locoregional therapies (catheter-based therapies and SBRT) and sorafenib are not considered curative. Although these therapies are often associated with durable responses, they have to be considered as a means to control HCC and in some cases a means to downsize or bridge the patient to more definitive options such as LT.

Q10. Option C – Palliation.

There are multiple therapeutic modalities for HCC, which include surgical options [resection or LT] and ablative electrochemical therapies (e.g., radiofrequency ablation or ethanol injection). Non-ablative treatment includes catheter-based embolic therapies (e.g., chemoembolisation and radioembolisation) and non-catheter-based therapy such as stereotactic body radiotherapy (SBRT). Finally, systemic therapy in the current era comprises solely of sorafenib, a multikinase inhibitor, and is non-curative. These therapeutic modalities can be broadly classified by therapeutic intent of attempting to cure or control the tumour. Surgical and ablative therapies are performed with curative intent, while the majority of locoregional therapies (catheter-based therapies and SBRT) and sorafenib are not considered curative. Although these therapies are often associated with durable responses, they have to be considered as a means to control HCC and in some cases a means to downsize or bridge the patient to more definitive options such as LT.

Q11. Option E – Diagnostic laparoscopy.

Postoperative bile leakage after laparoscopic cholecystectomy occurs in 1%–3% of cases. In patients undergoing day-case surgery, recovery is expected to be rapid and uncomplicated so any signs of intra-abdominal sepsis must be investigated urgently. Although a CT scan is often performed as a first-line investigation, in patients with signs of sepsis and peritonitis it would be safe to proceed direct to relook laparoscopy so that both diagnosis and treatment of the cause of deterioration can occur quickly. Ultrasound is not accurate enough in the postoperative period. After adequate peritoneal toilet and biliary drainage have been established, ERCP may be needed in case of persistent bile leakage. In cases of suspected bile duct injury, further imaging workup including contrast-enhanced CT, including arterial phase, and MRCP will help determine the site and nature of the injury.

Q12. Option E – Perform a palliative biliary decompression such as a percutaneous or endoscopic biliary stent placement.

Hilar cholangiocarcinoma (HCA) is the most common biliary tract malignancy and the second most common primary hepatic malignancy. It is classified into intrahepatic (iCCA), perihilar (pCCA), and distal (dCCA) subtypes. Inflammation and cholestasis are key factors in cholangiocarcinogenesis. Resectability for HCA is defined by the ability to completely remove the disease with curative intent while leaving an adequate liver remnant. A biopsy is not necessary if the surgeon suspects HCA and is planning curative resection. A biopsy should be obtained to confirm the diagnosis in the setting of unresectable disease. Assessment of resectability and/or intra- and extrahepatic metastatic disease, as well as venous and arterial invasion, is best accomplished using radiographic studies such as CT and/or MRI. Negative-margin (R0) resection rates can approach 85% with an aggressive surgical approach that often involves a major or extended hepatectomy. Therefore, intrahepatic cholangiocarcinoma is usually treated by hepatic resection, perihilar Klatskin tumour (bile duct and hepatic resection) and tumours of the distal bile duct require either a pancreaticoduodenectomy or less commonly, a local bile duct excision. The role of OTC for HCA remains controversial with a high incidence of lymph node metastasis. In this case, the disease is deemed unresectable and a palliative decompression approach should be adopted.

Criteria for unresectability in hilar cholangiocarcinoma:
1. Medically unfit patients
2. Distant metastatic disease – non-satellite hepatic metastases, lymph node metastases beyond portal vein, hepatic artery, coeliac axis and peripancreatic distribution
3. Extensive local involvement – bilateral or contralateral involvement of portal vein, hepatic artery or secondary biliary radicals
4. Inadequate future liver remnant – <30% FLR with normal (non-atrophied) hepatic parenchyma and adequate vascular inflow, outflow and biliary drainage

Criteria for unresectability in distal cholangiocarcinoma

Type 1

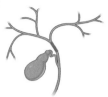

Tumour below the confluence of the right and left hepatic ducts

Type 2

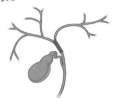

Tumour reaching the confleunce

Type 3a

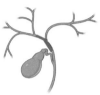

Tumour occluding the common hepatic and right hepatic duct

Type 3b

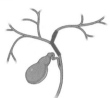

Tumour occluding the common hepatic and left hepatic duct

Type 4

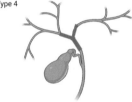

Tumour involves the confluence and both the right and left hepatic ducts

FIGURE 6.1   Types Bismuth-Corlette classification.

1. Medically unfit patients
2. Distant metastatic disease – liver and other organs; lymph node metastases beyond portal vein, hepatic artery, peripancreatic and coeliac axis distribution
3. Major vascular involvement – significant portal/superior mesenteric vein, superior mesenteric artery, common or proper hepatic artery

Bismuth-Corlette Classification of biliary tract cancers

Q13. Option E: Rouviere's sulcus is a fissure on the liver that corresponds to the level of the porta hepatis and dissection below this level is safe.

The critical view of safety is a "window" crossed by two structures: the cystic duct and artery only. Anterior and posterior dissection at the Hartman's pouch (alternating between inferolateral and supermedial retraction). The lower one-third of the gallbladder is separated from the liver to expose the cystic plate. The

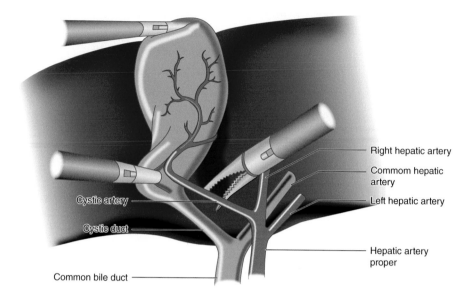

FIGURE 6.2   Critical view of safety.

critical view of safety should be achieved prior to clipping or dividing any tubular structures in laparoscopic cholecystectomy. Difficulty with the identification of the critical view should lead the surgeon to consider performing cholangiography or converting to an open procedure. Rouviere's sulcus is a fissure on the liver between the right lobe and caudate process and corresponds to the level of the porta hepatis. All dissection should be kept to a level above (or anterior) this sulcus to reduce the risk of injury to the bile duct.

A critical view of safety in laparoscopic cholecystectomy

Laparoscopic cholecystectomy steps:
1.   Accessing the abdomen
2.   Port placement
3.   Initial dissection of adhesions
4.   Dissection of the hepatocystic triangle
5.   Dissection of gallbladder off bottom one-third of the cystic plate
6.   Confirmation of critical view of safety
7.   Intraoperative cholangiogram if indicated
8.   Division of cystic duct and cystic artery
9.   Dissection of gallbladder off the remainder of the cystic plate
10.   Gallbladder extraction and port closure

Requirements of the critical view of safety:
1.   Clearance of hepatocystic triangle of all adipose and fibrous tissue

2. Removal of the gallbladder from the bottom one-third of the cystic plate of the liver
3. Two structures only seen entering the gallbladder: the cystic duct and cystic artery

If the critical view of safety cannot be obtained open cholecystectomy or subtotal fenestrating cholecystectomy should be considered

Q14. Option D – CT-guided drainage of intra-abdominal fluid collection and transfer to a tertiary HPB Centre.

The incidence of bile duct injury following laparoscopic cholecystectomy has been estimated to be 0.15%–0.3% of all cases. The goal of treatment is to eradicate the transpapillary pressure gradient thereby allowing the free flow of bile. The decision for the type of treatment depends on a range of factors comprising the severity of the patient's presentation and Strasberg's classification of the injury.

Strasberg Classification of iatrogenic bile duct injury:

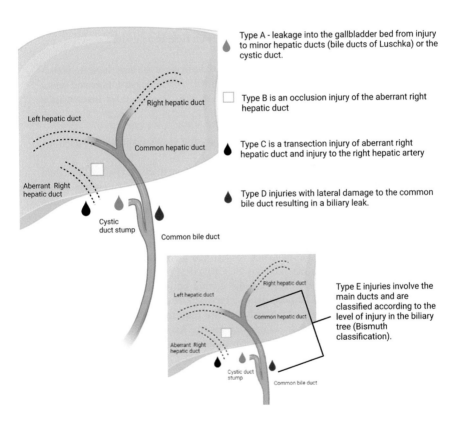

FIGURE 6.3   Strasberg Classification of iatrogenic bile duct injury.

Type A involves leakage into the gallbladder bed from injury to minor hepatic ducts (bile ducts of Luschka) or the cystic duct. Management ERCP and stent placement. Type B is an occlusion injury of the aberrant right hepatic duct. The patient may remain asymptomatic for years and then present with right upper quadrant pain, and fever due to recurrent cholangitis and segmental fibrosis and/or atrophy may result. Diagnosis is made by ERCP (absent of segmental hepatic duct) and treatment is surgical resection of the affected lobe with hepaticojejunostomy. Type C is a transection injury of the aberrant right hepatic duct and injury to the right hepatic artery is a common association. Type D injuries with lateral damage to the CBD resulting in a biliary leak. Management for type C and D injuries can be managed with an ERCP sphincterotomy / stent. Type E injuries involve the main ducts and are classified according to the level of injury in the biliary tree (Bismuth classification). The most common reconstruction for proximal bile duct injury is Roux-en-Y hepaticojejunostomy.

- E1 (Bismuth type 1) Injury more than 2 cm from the confluence
- E2 (Bismuth type 2) Injury less than 2 cm from the confluence
- E3 (Bismuth type 3) Injury at the confluence; confluence intact
- E4 (Bismuth type 4) Destruction of the biliary confluence
- E5 (Bismuth type 5) Injury to the aberrant right hepatic duct

In the above scenario, external percutaneous drainage of the large loculated intra-abdominal collection with a catheter left in will avoid bile peritonitis and sepsis source control. The modality (ERCP versus MRCP) chosen for investigation depends on the suspected injury pattern.

Q15. Option C – Diagnostic laparoscopy and proceed to extended cholecystectomy with wedge resection of segment 4B/5.

Gallbladder adenocarcinoma has an overall median survival of less than 6 months and spreads early to distant organs. Patients are often asymptomatic but can present with abdominal pain and weight loss. Obstructive jaundice is an ominous sign with a poor prognosis. It should be emphasised that a tissue diagnosis is not necessary prior to surgical exploration. Absolute contraindications to resection are liver, peritoneal metastasis, malignant ascites, encasement or occlusion of major vessels and locoregional metastatic lymph node disease. Tumour extends into the CBD, or a negative cystic duct margin (as determined by the frozen section) cannot be obtained, extrahepatic bile duct resection should be performed. T1aN0M0 disease is presumed cured by simple cholecystectomy alone and does not require liver resection. However, for T3 tumours that have direct invasion into the liver bed, a formal resection of segment 4b/5 is recommended as a substitute for wedge resection.

Q16. Option B – Perform ERCP/EUS to further characterise the cyst.

Choledochal cysts are biliary malformations that are classified according to the site (extrahepatic or intrahepatic), shape (saccular or fusiform) and extent (segmental or complete throughout the biliary tree). They are associated with complications such as cholangitis, pancreatitis, ductal stones and stricture formation and a high risk of malignancy.

There are six types of choledochal malformations described by Todani:

- Type I: Fusiform dilation of the CBD, the most common type of cyst, high risk of malignancy and surgical management is advised (cysts completely removed with Roux-en-Y hepaticojejunostomy).
- Type II: True extrahepatic bile duct diverticulum, 2% of cysts, if they become symptomatic then management with simple cyst excision resection in the absence of neoplasia.

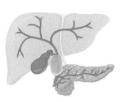

Type I: Fusiform dilation of the common bile duct

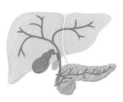

Type II: True extrahepatic bile duct diverticulum

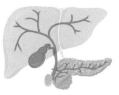

Type III: Intraduodenal saccular dilation of the common bile duct in the ampulla

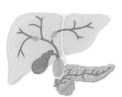

Type IVA: Intra- and extrahepatic cysts

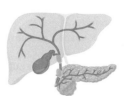

Type IVB: Extrahepatic cysts only

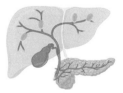

Type V: Multiple cystic dilation of the intrahepatic bile ducts,

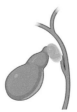

Type VI: Isolated cystic dilations of the cyst duct.

FIGURE 6.4   Types of choledochal malformations.

- Type III: Intraduodenal saccular dilation of the CBD in the ampulla, termed choledochocele. Management with ERCP sphincterotomy or endoscopic resection is recommended.
- Type IV: Multiple cystic bile duct dilations, the second most common type of cyst.
- Type IVA: Intra- and extrahepatic cysts
- Type IVB: Extrahepatic cysts only
- NB: Intrahepatic type IV cysts: undergo partial hepatectomy for excision of the intrahepatic portion of the cyst and reconstruction with wide hilar Roux-en-Y hepaticojejunostomy.
- Type V: Multiple fusiform or saccular cystic dilation of the intrahepatic bile ducts, whether or not associated with hepatic fibrosis (Caroli disease). These can be difficult to manage and some patients require LT.
- Type VI: Isolated cystic dilations of the cyst duct. If there is a narrow connection to the CBD, then cyst excision and cholecystectomy are recommended. However, if the cyst is in continuity with the CBD then a hepaticojejunostomy is performed.

Biliary cysts are associated with an increased risk of cancer, particularly cholangiocarcinoma and are frequently found in the posterior cyst wall. The incidence of malignancy increases with age. For patients with type 1 or IV cysts, complete cyst excision and Roux-en-Y hepaticojejunostomy are recommended. The current "gold standard" for staging is an MRI pancreas/MRCP to visualise the biliary tree followed by a EUS/ERCP that will allow direct visualisation of the ampulla and pancreatic duct.

Q17. Option C – Initial management consists of supportive care with fluid resuscitation, pain control and nutritional support.

As per the Atlanta classification, acute pancreatitis can be divided into two categories:
- Interstitial oedematous acute pancreatitis, inflammation of the pancreatic parenchyma and peripancreatic tissues, no tissue necrosis.
- Necrotising acute pancreatitis, inflammation associated with pancreatic parenchymal necrosis and/or peripancreatic necrosis.

WON (walled-off necrosis) is an established, encapsulated collection of necrosis that has developed an inflammatory wall. WON>4weeks after onset of necrotising pancreatitis.

A CT severity score (the Balthazar score) has been developed based on the degree of necrosis, inflammation, and the presence of fluid collections

CT severity index (Table 6.1)

According to the severity, acute pancreatitis is divided into the following:
- Mild acute pancreatitis – no organ failure and local or systemic complications – Balthazar B or C
- Moderately severe acute pancreatitis, which is characterised by no or transient organ failure (<48hours) and/or local complications – Balthazar D or E
- Severe acute pancreatitis, persistent organ failure (>48hours) that may involve one or multiple organs

Initial management consists of supportive care with fluid resuscitation, pain control and nutritional support. Enteral feeding rather than parenteral nutrition

TABLE 6.1
Grading Based on Unenhanced CT Findings

Grade	Findings	Score
A	Normal pancreas – normal size, sharply defined, smooth contour, homogenous enhancement, retroperitoneal peripancreatic fat, fat without enhancement	0
B	Focal or diffuse enlargement of the pancreas, the contour may show irregularity, enhancement may be inhomogeneous, but there is no peripancreatic inflammation	1
C	Peripancreatic inflammation with intrinsic pancreatic abnormalities	2
D	Intrapancreatic or extrapancreatic fluid collections	3
E	2 or more collections of gas in the pancreas or retroperitoneum	4
Necrosis based on contrast-enhanced CT(%)		
0%		0
<33%		2
33%–50%		4
≥50%		6

is recommended in patients with moderately severe and severe acute pancreatitis who cannot tolerate oral feeding. Treatment should focus on underlying pancreatitis as effective treatment may result in spontaneous resolution of the thrombosis. However, anticoagulation is recommended if there is a thrombosis extending into the portal or superior mesenteric vein, leading to a compromise in hepatic function or bowel perfusion.

Q18. Option B – Endoscopic cyst gastrostomy, fully covered, self-expandable metal stent.

Acute pancreatitis is a potentially fatal condition and 20% of patients will develop pancreatic necrosis of those will have mortality is 30%. Minimally invasive pancreatic necrosectomy is the gold standard of management for pancreatic necrosis requiring intervention.

In stable patients with infected necrosis, advice is to delay intervention for at least 4 weeks with conservative management. This will allow the necrotic material to mature and become more amenable to minimally invasive debridement. PANTER trial has shown a step-up approach (endoscopic and percutaneous drainage) to be more beneficial for patients compared to an open necrosectomy that has high morbidity and mortality. Postponed or immediate drainage of infected necrotising pancreatitis (POINTER trial) did not show the superiority of immediate catheter drainage when compared with postponed catheter drainage. However, hybrid utilisation of all available techniques remains integral to optimal outcomes.

A step-up approach for necrotising pancreatitis:

First step:
- Percutaneous or endoscopic transgastric drainage
- Left retroperitoneal approach 93%, transabdominal 2% and endoscopic 5%
Second step (if there is no clinical improvement after 72 hours)
- Drain repositioning or second drain insertion
Third step (if there is no clinical improvement after 72 hours)
- Video-assisted retroperitoneal debridement (VARD)

The Dutch pancreatic group reported that infected necrosis was confirmed on positive fine needle aspiration (FNA) in 86% of cases, gas on CT imaging in 94% and clinical symptoms in 80% (p=0.07). They concluded that diagnosis can be made on clinical or imaging signs of infection and FNA may be useful in patients with unclear clinical/imaging signs.

A multicentre randomised trial demonstrated that an endoscopic step-up approach was not superior to a surgical step-up approach in reducing major complications and death from pancreatic necrosis. However, Van Brunschot *et al.* reported reduced pancreatic fistula rates, length of hospital stays and lower costs with the endoscopic approach. There were no patients requiring open necrosectomy, and 40% were treated with endoscopic drainage only, while 51% were treated with CT-guided drainage only.

Q19. Option A – ERCP and metal-covered stent.

Pancreatic ductal adenocarcinoma (PDAC) is a lethal disease. PDAC has a particularly poor overall prognosis, with a 5-year overall survival (OS) of just 9%, largely due to the fact that most patients present with advanced-stage disease and most treatment regimens are ineffective. Even when patients can undergo surgical resection, the recurrence rate is very high and the median OS varies between 24 and 30 months. The role of pre-operative biliary drainage (PBD) before surgery for tumours of the pancreatic head causing biliary obstruction has been controversial. However, patients who are deeply jaundiced are at risk for perioperative complications and were found to be a worse prognostic factor for OS after surgery. Shen *et al.* proposed that PBD has an important role in severely jaundiced patients (bilirubin ≥ 250 µmol/L). Malnutrition is common in patients with obstructive jaundice and PBD has been shown to improve food intake in patients with malignant biliary obstruction. Whereas, the 2012 Cochrane review (six RCTs) comparing PBD and direct to found no significant difference in the rate of mortality or serious morbidity between the two intervention groups. In practice, jaundiced patients may have already undergone biliary stenting before resectability or the time frame for resection has been determined. A severely obstructive jaundice patient should undergo pre-operative drainage and ERCP with a stent is the preferred method. PTC drainage is reserved for cases of ERCP failure.

Q20. Option C – Refer for neoadjuvant chemotherapy.

Locally advanced pancreatic cancer (LAPC) is a non-metastasised pancreatic cancer, in which upfront resection is considered not beneficial due to extensive vascular involvement and a consequent high chance of a non-radical resection.

Society of Surgical Oncology/American Hepato-Pancreato-Biliary Association/ National Comprehensive Cancer Network (NCCN) guidelines for the criteria of borderline resectability are:

- No distant metastases
- Venous involvement of the SMV/PV with or without impingement and narrowing of the lumen
- Short segment venous occlusion but with suitable vessel proximal and distal length to allow safe resection and reconstruction
- Gastroduodenal artery (GDA) encasement up to the hepatic artery (HA)
- Tumour contact with SMA is not to exceed 180° of the circumference
- Tumour contact with the common hepatic artery without extension to the celiac axis or hepatic artery bifurcation
- For tumours of the body/tail – tumour contact with the celiac axis of ≤180 degrees, if >180 degrees then without the involvement of the aorta or GDA

Management of LAPC is in evolution, with the majority of these patients undergoing neoadjuvant therapy. Studies have shown that patients that have had omission of neoadjuvant therapy are associated with early disease reoccurrence, early treatment of micro-metastatic disease, higher margin-negative resection (R0) rates and optimised delivery of systemic therapy. A tissue diagnosis is required before the initiation of neoadjuvant therapy if planned.

Q21. Option A – Colorectal first approach.

Surgical resection is the only curative method for Colorectal liver metastasis (CRLM) and an R0 resection margin is the ultimate goal. Operative planning should be based on maintaining inflow (hepatic artery and portal vein), outflow (hepatic veins), biliary drainage and adequate future liver reserve to prevent post-hepatectomy liver failure. Within this scenario, a "colorectal first approach" should be performed. The patient has presented with symptoms from their primary colorectal cancer such as impending perforation and obstruction and will require an emergency ultra-low Hartmann's. Once he has recovered from surgery, systemic chemotherapy should be offered prior to CRLM resection. The reverse (liver-first) approach starts with chemotherapy first, liver surgery second, and performing colorectal surgery last. This avoids the risk of metastatic progression during the treatment of the primary tumour. Simultaneous resection can be performed for favourable colonic tumours (right hemicolectomy) and minor liver resection. Extensive disease should not be managed simultaneously. When simultaneous resection is performed, the liver resection is performed first. Patients with extensive bilobar diseases would benefit from a two-staged approach: at the time of colorectal primary resection, minor wedge CRLMs are resected, leaving tumours behind on the part of the liver that will be treated with a future anatomic resection. The patient then undergoes portal vein embolisation on the side with the remaining tumours, allowing an increase in the future remnant liver. Then, a formal anatomic resection can be performed on the tumour side.

Q22. Option B – Duodenal stenting.

Palliative treatment of malignancy gastric outlet obstruction includes endoscopic placement of self-expanding metal stents and surgical gastrojejunostomy. In patients with good performance status, both methods are associated with good technical success rates, although recovery following stenting is often faster. It is reasonable to consider duodenal stenting as a first-line option, with surgical gastrojejunostomy as a second-line treatment. In patients with poor performance status, palliation may be appropriate and should be carefully discussed with the patient and their relatives. Survival after duodenal stenting is usually measured in months.

Q23. Option C – right hepatic artery.

25% of people will have either a replaced or accessory right hepatic artery, running laterally to the portal vein. This is at risk of injury in laparoscopic cholecystectomy. Post-mortem examination of patients who had undergone cholecystectomy but died of other causes showed the incidence of unrecognised injury of the right hepatic artery is 7%, and the incidence of right hepatic artery injury in patients with bile duct injuries is between 10% and 40%.

Q24. Option D – MRCP.

This patient has signs of biliary sepsis and a known history of gallstones. While ultrasound is often the first-line investigation of all patients, this patient has already had ultrasound-confirmed gallstones. Therefore, the investigation is directed towards determining if there are CBD stones, which can be assessed most accurately by MRCP. USS diagnosis of ductal stones is less accurate, especially in patients with obesity and ionising radiation in younger patients should be minimised if possible. Although ERCP may be required, the risk of complications is at least 5% so ERCP should be reserved for those patients with definite CBD stones. Proceeding directly to surgery without further investigation may occur in some specialist centres but, in general, the pre-operative investigation will help to plan surgical intervention and is recommended by BSG guidelines.

Q25. Option E – Repeat ultrasound scan in 12 months.

Gallbladder polyps >10 mm in diameter are associated with >1% risk of malignancy and cholecystectomy should be offered to patients fit for surgery. Even so, >70% of ultrasonically identified gallbladder polyps are actually stones. Therefore, patients with polyps and typical biliary symptoms may be offered surgery. Ultrasound remains the most sensitive method of assessing the gallbladder for sludge and small stones, and therefore axial imaging with CT and MRI is not usually helpful. In cases where USS accuracy is doubted, a second ultrasound scan by an experienced sonographer is appropriate.

In an attempt to rationalise follow-up, ESGAR 2017 guidelines identify the following as risk factors for malignancy – Age>50 years, history of primary sclerosing cholangitis, Indian ethnicity, sessile polyp (with focal wall thickening>4 mm). Patients with polyps 6–9 mm in diameter can have surveillance scans at 6 months and then yearly for a total of 5 years. Patients with polyp<6 mm should be offered USS at 1, 3 and 5 years. If during follow-up, the polyp grows by 2 mm or more, reaches 10 mm in size or the patient develops biliary symptoms, surgery should be offered.

Q26. Option C – Refer to hepatobiliary surgeon for consideration of liver resection – wedge resection or formal Sg IVb/V resection.

Gallbladder cancer presents in two main ways – incidental histology finding in patients undergoing cholecystectomy for symptomatic gallstones and gallbladder mass. The prognosis is poor and surgical resection is associated with the best survival outcomes. T1a tumours limited to the lamina propria, or foci of dysplasia or carcinoma in situ are sufficiently treated by cholecystectomy alone. T1b and above should be offered liver resection of the gallbladder bed (either through non-anatomical wedge resection or formal segmental resection) along with lymphadenectomy. Involvement of the cystic duct margin necessitates excision of the extrahepatic biliary tree and hepaticojejunostomy.

Gallbladder cancer is poorly sensitive to radiotherapy and very effective chemotherapy regimens have not been established. Although it did not reach its primary end-point criteria, the BILCAP trial (2019) has shown that adjuvant capecitabine for resected biliary tract cancers is associated with improved survival compared with observation alone. ABC-02 trial (2010) showed that a combination of gemcitabine and cisplatin is associated with a modest survival advantage over gemcitabine alone in patients with metastatic biliary cancers.

Due to poor overall outcomes, even in patients undergoing radical resection, the Newcastle HPB Unit proposed a "delayed staging" strategy, in an effort to select out patients with rapidly progressive disease using a "test of time". This is in contrast to "fast track" gallbladder bed resection, which was supported by French registry data. Despite comparable outcomes and reduced rates of R1 resection, at present, this delayed staging strategy is not widely practised.

Q27. Option B – PET scan followed by pancreaticoduodenectomy.

Survival outcomes in patients with pancreatic cancer remain poor and radical surgical resection remains the best treatment, in selected patients. Urgent investigation of patients presenting with obstructive jaundice is aimed

1. Treating sepsis, dehydration and assessing nutrition
2. Determining a cause, especially excluding gallstones
3. If a tumour is suspected, excluding obvious metastases, especially in the liver
4. Confirming suitability for surgery – including resectability of tumour/extent of local advancement

In the presence of cholangitis and biliary obstruction, biliary decompression via ERCP or PTC is necessary. However, if there is no sepsis, patients may benefit from proceeding directly to surgery. A randomised trial of PBD before PD (Dutch trial, NEJM 2010) showed that in patients with bilirubin <250, there were fewer complications in the no-drainage group.

The PET PANC study upstaged 20% of patients planned for PD and therefore is a cost-effective and important additional investigation in patients with potentially resectable pancreatic cancer.

Q28. Option E – Laparoscopic non-anatomical segment 6 resection.

In the setting of colorectal cancer surveillance, new liver lesions can be presumed to be metastases. Liver biopsy should be avoided, due to the risk of seeding and procedure-related complications, and add no additional diagnostic benefit (with potentially reduced survival). The New EPOC trials showed a small disease-free survival benefit at 3 years in patients who have neoadjuvant chemotherapy, although there was no overall 5-year survival benefit. Advantages of a neo-adjuvant approach include downstaging to make resection easier or improve the R0 rate, and as a "test of time" to select out rapidly progressive disease where liver resection would be of little prognostic benefit.

Liver resection remains the optimal treatment for colorectal liver metastases. Multiple series report >50% 5-year survival in selected patients undergoing surgery. Fifty per cent of patients with colorectal cancer will develop metastases but at present, <15% have disease amenable to liver resection. In this patient, favourable prognostic factors include solitary metastases and metachronous disease (i.e. presenting >2 years from primary surgery). In any fit patient, surgery should be considered and there is a strong recommendation in the UK that all colorectal cancer MDTs should include a liver surgeon as a core member.

The techniques of liver surgery have evolved over the last 30 years so that the extent of possible resection has increased, while mortality and morbidity have decreased. Repeated liver resections are associated with long postoperative survival. Parenchymal sparing surgery is increasingly favoured as long as a clear resection margin can be obtained – there is no advantage of >1 mm margin, so hemihepatectomy for solitary metastases is only required for very large lesions or in cases where vascular inflow and/or outflow is threatened by the tumour. Laparoscopic liver surgery is increasingly common, with the indications also extending as techniques and experience improve. The usual advantages of laparoscopy, such as decreased length of stay and fewer hernias, are preserved.

Q29. Option C – Emergency exploratory laparotomy + proceed.

Perforation occurs in approximately ~0.5% of ERCP. Stapfer classification is type I, lateral or medial wall duodenal perforation; type II, peri-vaterian injuries; type III, distal bile duct injuries related to guidewire-basket instrumentation and type IV, retroperitoneal air alone.

ERCP reports contain the key information in terms of predicting what has happened. Usually, with type 1 injuries, the endoscopist finds it difficult to insufflate and will notice (and document) the perforation. In type III and IV injuries, usually, the procedure is uneventful and only noted afterwards. In this case, because wire-guided access was not possible, a small incision had to be made at the presumed papilla. As this is essentially a "freehand" technique, any deviation from the correct line may result in a medial duodenal wall injury. This may have been compounded by inserting a stent through the enterotomy.

Patients with signs of sepsis/septic shock need urgent fluid resuscitation, intravenous antibiotics and ideally source control. Although laparoscopy may be useful in certain situations, the safest choice is to proceed with open surgery. In this situation, washout of the infected fluid, along with aggressive drainage of the right upper quadrant is an appropriate initial procedure. As the patient is unwell, the priority is source control, and more definitive management can be deferred, including transfer to a specialist centre if needed.

Q30. Option C – Creatinine.

Child-Pugh score was originally developed to assess the severity of chronic liver disease due to cirrhosis; however, its use has been widened since its description in 1964. It includes clinical as well as lab parameters including ascites, encephalopathy, INR/prolonged PT, bilirubin and albumin. Each parameter is given a score of 1 to 3 depending upon the values and a total score is calculated to define Child's Class. Higher scores indicate worsening liver function, liver comorbidity and liver reserves. This score is also used in predicting perioperative mortality and guiding the treatment of HCC (Table 6.2). Model for End-stage Liver Disease (MELD) uses bilirubin, creatinine and INR.

TABLE 6.2
Cirrhosis Mortality by Class

Cirrhosis Class	Score	Mortality
A	5–6 points	10%
B	7–9 points	30%
C	10–15 points	70%–80%

Q31. Option A – CBD.

The free edge of the lesser of lesser omentum between the stomach and liver is thin and fragile, and it contains a bile duct on the right and a hepatic artery on the left, both lying anterior to the portal vein. The CBD is most vulnerable at this place and likely to be injured during laparoscopic cholecystectomy. It is also a site to perform the Pringle manoeuvre (occlusion of the main portal pedicle). Many other risk factors have been included that increase the risks of bile duct injury during laparoscopic cholecystectomy including acute cholecystitis, bleeding in Calot's triangle, severely scarred or shrunken gall bladder, largely impacted gallstone in Hartmann's pouch, short cystic duct, Mirizzi's syndrome and abnormal biliary anatomy.

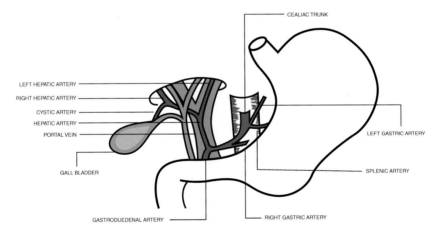

FIGURE 6.5

Q32. Option C – Superior mesenteric artery.

The liver receives a dual blood supply from the portal vein (75%) and hepatic artery (25%). The hepatic artery, classically present in approximately 76% of cases, takes its origin from the celiac trunk and divides into the right and left hepatic arteries. In approximately 10%–15% of the cases, the replaced or accessory hepatic artery arises from the superior mesenteric artery which travels posterior to the portal vein and then takes up the right lateral position before diving into the liver parenchyma. In approximately 3%–10% of cases, there exists a replacement or accessory left hepatic artery coming off of the left gastric artery and running obliquely in the gastrohepatic ligament anterior to the caudate lobe before entering into the liver.

Q33. Option B – Left hepatic vein.

    The liver drains into IVC usually by three large veins namely right, left and middle hepatic veins. The right hepatic vein can be exposed fully outside the liver before it joins IVC below the diaphragm. The left and middle hepatic veins unite within the liver parenchyma to form a common channel before entering into the IVC.

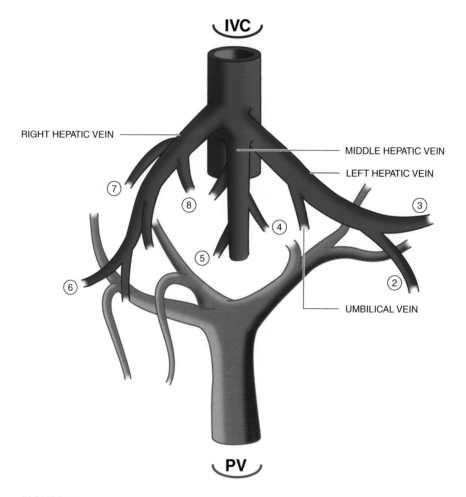

FIGURE 6.6

Q34. Option A – Large pancreatic duct diameter.

    Postoperative pancreatic fistula remains a serious postoperative complication in procedures involving the pancreas including pancreatic resections, splenectomy and gastrectomy. The ISGPF (2016) classifies pancreatic fistulas into three categories as shown in Table 6.3.

TABLE 6.3
POPF Grading System

Grade	Definition
Biochemical leakage (BL)	Drainage amylase >3 times the upper limit institutional normal serum amylase value and no clinical impact.
Grade B	Persistent drainage >3 weeks, clinically relevant change in management of POPF, percutaneous or endoscopic drainage, angiographic procedures for bleeding, signs of infection without organ failure.
Grade C	Reoperation, organ failure or death.

For pancreatoduodenectomy, small duct size; soft gland texture; ampullary, duodenal, cystic, or islet cell pathology; and increased intraoperative blood loss are convincing risk factors for the development of clinically relevant fistulae as judged by ISGPF classification. In some studies, a pancreatic duct size of >3 mm is associated with an increased incidence of pancreatic fistula. Other risk factors include older age, obesity, and pulmonary or renal comorbidity. Procedure-related factors include prolonged operating time and the need for blood transfusion, vascular or multi-visceral resections, type of anastomosis, or pancreatic stump closure and stent use.

Q35. Option C – To institute neoadjuvant therapy.

Surgical resection (Whipple's procedure or pylorus-preserving pancreaticoduodenectomy) combined with adjuvant chemotherapy remains the mainstay of treatment of pancreatic head cancers. Neoadjuvant chemotherapy or chemoradiotherapy is considered in patients with borderline resectable tumours e.g., with early involvement of portal vein or other vascular structures. This group of patients may benefit from PBD. Biliary intervention (ERCP/ PTC) is to be avoided before MDM discussion as optimum treatment may be compromised through the introduction of infection or procedure-related morbidity. Other reasons for biliary drainage include optimisation of the quality of life through the relief of obstructive symptoms and pain control in a selected group of patients.

Q36. Option E – Technetium-99m colloid scan.

Tc-99m RBC scintigraphy is a noninvasive method, which provides the most specific diagnosis of hepatic hemangioma. The characteristic, diagnostic presentation of HH on Tc-99-labelled RBC images is perfusion/blood pool mismatch: decreased perfusion on early dynamic images and a gradual increase in activity on blood pool images over time. The lesion appears "cold" in the early dynamic phase and finally intense in the late phase, 1–2 hours following Tc-99m injection. Sensitivity is strongly size-dependent, especially at the small end of the range: 17%–20% for the detection of lesions less than 1 cm in size, 65%–80% for lesions between 1 and 2 cm, and virtually 100% for those larger than 2 cm. The specificity of Tc-99m labelled RBC scintigraphy with single-photon emission CT remains at 100% over the entire size range. Although it has very high sensitivity and specificity, scintigraphy is always followed by either a CT or a US exam to establish the location, shape and multiplicity of the lesion.

Q37. Option B – Serous cystadenoma.

Overall, the risk of malignancy in incidentally detected pancreatic cysts is low. A technical review from the American Gastroenterological Association estimated that the risk of malignancy in a pancreatic cyst at the time of diagnosis is at most 0.01% (0.21% for cysts >2 cm). In the subset of cysts that were surgically resected, it was found that the risk of malignancy was 15%. However, there is significant selection bias in the surgical series in which cysts were resected. Factors associated with an increased risk of malignancy included cyst size >3 cm (43% versus 22% if the cyst was <3 cm, odds ratio [OR] 3.0) and finding a solid component within the cyst (73% versus 23% if there was no solid component, OR 7.7). There was a trend towards an increased risk of malignancy if the main pancreatic duct was dilated (47% versus 33% if the duct was not dilated, OR 2.4, 95% CI 0.7–8.0). There was no association between the risk of malignancy and cyst enlargement over time.

In addition to the above factors, the malignant potential of a cyst also depends on the cyst type. Serous cystic tumours are at very low risk for developing malignancy, whereas the risk is moderate to high in mucinous cystic neoplasms, solid pseudopapillary tumours and some intraductal papillary mucinous tumours of the pancreas (intraductal papillary mucinous neoplasms (IPMNs); up to 70% for main-duct IPMNs).

Q38. Option C – Use of prophylactic antibiotics.

The majority of patients with acute pancreatitis resolve with conservative management alone, however, around 15%–20% of the cases develop multisystem illness potentially leading to organ failure. This group of patients are usually managed in ITU settings. Studies have revealed that the preferred approach includes pain relief, fluid therapy, enteral nutrition support, intensive organ support and a step-up intervention for pancreatic necrosis. There is no role for use of prophylactic antibiotics in preventing mortality in cases of severe acute pancreatitis. Early use of antibiotics is only indicated in cases of suspected or proven cholangitis while waiting for urgent ERCP.

Q39. Option C – Ligation of left hepatic duct.

Bile duct injuries following laparoscopic cholecystectomy may present as features of obstructive jaundice. Various risk factors have been identified in the literature with include bile leaks, injury/ligation of CBD, CHD and right hepatic duct, stones in CBD and rarely external compression from biloma. While all other options could be the cause of obstructive jaundice, ligation of the left hepatic duct is a very unlikely event to occur while performing laparoscopic cholecystectomy.

Q40. Option D – Bite cells.

Howell-Jolly bodies are abnormal cytoplasmic inclusions of basophilic nuclear remnants within RBCs which are normally removed by a functioning spleen. Target cells are altered RBCs which are removed by the spleen as well. Echinocytes, also known as blur cells, are a form of RBCs with abnormal cell membranes characterised by many small projections. Pappenheimer bodies are abnormal granules of iron found inside RBCs as inclusion bodies formed by phagosomes. Bite cells are abnormally shaped mature red blood cells which result from the mechanical removal of denatured haemoglobin during splenic filtration.

Q41. Option E – Atelectasis.

Perioperative complications of open splenectomy may be classified as pulmonary, haemorrhagic (intraoperative and postoperative), infectious (subphrenic abscess and wound infection), pancreatic (pancreatitis, pseudocyst and pancreatic fistula) and thromboembolic. Left lower lobe atelectasis is the most common complication after open splenectomy; pleural effusion and pneumonia also can occur.

Q42. Option E – ARDS.

The incidence of acute pancreatitis is in the range of 300 or more patients per million annually. Using the Atlanta classification on severity, about 10% of acute pancreatitis patients are classified as severe. About one-third of all deaths from acute pancreatitis have been reported to occur prior to admission to the hospital, and in most cases, is associated with acute lung injury (ALI). Hospital deaths occur within the first week after admission in 35%–50% and the cause of death is related to single or multiple organ failure in a majority of cases. In elderly patients, up to 60% of all deaths within the first week are considered to be caused by pancreatitis-associated ALI and acute respiratory distress syndrome (ARDS). Independently, ALI is a consequence of a pronounced systemic inflammatory response with increased endothelial and epithelial barrier permeability, with leakage of a protein-rich exudate into the alveolar space and interstitial tissues, thus compromising oxygenation and gas exchange. The magnitude of the systemic inflammatory response determines the concomitant clinical course and outcome, and this also is true for the severity of the acute-pancreatitis-associated ALI. Respiratory complications are frequent in acute pancreatitis, and respiratory dysfunction, presenting as ALI or ARDS, is a major component of multiple organ dysfunction syndromes, with a frequent need for ventilatory support, which contributes to early death in severe acute pancreatitis

Q43. Option D – Acute pancreatitis.

Pancreatitis due to medications is rare (<5%). However, proving the association with a particular drug may not always be straightforward, even in suspected cases. Pancreatitis may develop within a few weeks after beginning a drug associated with an immunologically mediated adverse reaction; in this setting, the patient may also have a rash and eosinophilia. In contrast, patients taking valproic acid or pentamidine may not develop pancreatitis until after many months of use, presumably due to the chronic accumulation of toxic metabolic products. Thus, patients restarted on their medications should be closely monitored and the drug promptly discontinued if symptoms recur. Most of the published evidence is based on case reports and, hence, it is very important to rule out all other causes before attributing a drug as the cause of acute pancreatitis.

Q44. Option A – Left triangular ligament.

The liver is covered in a thin fibrous capsule called Glisson's capsule. Numerous peritoneal reflections fix the liver in the right upper quadrant. Anterior and posterior folds of left triangular ligaments attach the superior surface of the left lobe of the liver with the diaphragm. Dividing these folds allows the left lobe to be mobilised from the diaphragm and the left lateral wall of the inferior vena cava (IVC) to be exposed. Division of the right triangular ligament allows the right lobe of the liver to be mobilised from under the diaphragm and rotated to the left. Division of the superior leaves of the falciform ligament (remnant of the umbilical vein which runs from the umbilicus to the interlobar fissure) allows exposure of the suprahepatic IVC, lying within a thin sheath of fibrous tissue. The lesser omentum (between the stomach and the liver) is often thin and fragile but contains the hilar structures in its free edge.

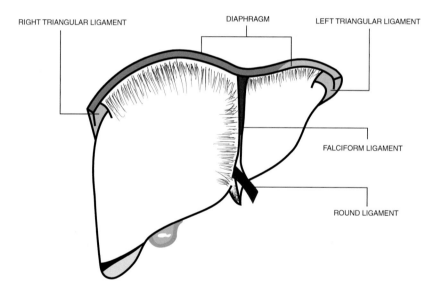

FIGURE 6.7

Q45. Option C – The Upper pole of the spleen is more commonly injured, owing to its orientation and the greater concentration of peritoneal attachments.

Intraoperative injury to the spleen has been linked with numerous operations, such as gastric fundoplication, colectomy, paraoesophageal hernia repair, nephrectomy, abdominal and pelvic vascular surgery and endoscopic procedures such as colonoscopy. Improper traction on the spleen against its peritoneal attachments is the most common mechanism of intraoperative injury. Capsular tears are the most common type of injury, but parenchymal lacerations and subcapsular hematomas also occur. The lower pole is more commonly injured, owing to its orientation and the greater concentration of peritoneal attachments found here. When dealing with capsular tears (the most common injury), strong consideration should be given to splenorrhaphy techniques: application of topical hemostatics, suture plication of disrupted parenchyma with or without omental buttress and the use of bioabsorbable mesh sheets.

Q46. Option E – All of the above.

Q47. Option D – Severe abdominal compartment syndrome.

Close monitoring of such patients by clinical examinations, inflammatory markers and cross-sectional images is required for optimal management and timely intervention. A pancreatic protocol CT scan is indicated for significant clinical deterioration and elevated CRP, suspicion of local pancreatic complications, suspected bowel ischaemia and acute bleeding (CT angiogram – if stable enough and consider embolisation and for abdominal compartment syndrome). Following the publication of a large Dutch randomised trial, a step-up approach for intervention has been widely accepted ad includes various minimally invasive techniques including percutaneous or endoscopic drainage. The open surgical approach is considered only after failure of minimally invasive techniques, acute abdomen (perforation/ischaemia) and severe abdominal compartment syndrome requiring open decompression.

Q48. Option D – Unresectable extrahepatic malignancy.

Resection of CRLM has been part of the routine treatment of colorectal cancer in modern surgical practice. Previously, patients with synchronous disease, rectal primary, multiple diffuse metastases, metastases larger than 5cm, a disease-free interval of less than 1 year from the diagnosis of the primary disease or a high serum carcinoembryonic antigen (CEA) were considered irresectable and suitable only for palliative treatment. However, since the publication of various studies in the last 20 years about the safety and efficacy of liver resection, the indications for hepatic resection now centre on what will remain after resection. A patient with a normal underlying liver requires at least a 20% FLR to prevent postoperative liver failure, 30% FLR for patients who have steatosis or steatohepatitis, often after receiving pre-operative chemotherapy, and 40% FLR in patients with underlying cirrhosis. Oncological contraindication includes unresectable extrahepatic malignancy e.g., CRC metastases to lungs, intra-abdominal lymph nodes and peritoneum. The use of neoadjuvant chemotherapy, portal vein embolisation, two-stage hepatectomy, simultaneous ablation, and resection of the extrahepatic tumour in select patients have increased the number of patients eligible for a surgical approach.

FURTHER READING

Al-Hawary MM, Francis IR, Chari ST, et al. Pancreatic ductal adenocarcinoma radiology reporting template: consensus statement of the Society of Abdominal Radiology and the American Pancreatic Association. *Radiology*. 2014;270:248.

Amarjothi JMV, Ramasamy V, Jesudasan J, NaganathBabu OL. Type VI choledochal cysts-case report and review of literature. *Surg J*. 2019;5(3):82–86.

Ammori JB, Colletti LM, Zalupski MM, et al. Surgical resection following radiation therapy with concurrent gemcitabine in patients with previously unresectable adenocarcinoma of the pancreas. *J Gastrointest Surg*. 2003;7:766.

Bajenaru N, Balaban V, Săvulescu F, Campeanu I, Patrascu T. Hepatic hemangioma -review. *J Med Life*. 2015;8 Spec Issue(Spec Issue):4–11.

Balthazar EJ, Robinson DL, Megibow AJ, Ranson JH. Acute pancreatitis: value of CT in establishing prognosis. *Radiology*. 1990;174:331.

Banks PA, Bollen TL, Dervenis C, et al. Classification of acute pancreatitis–2012: revision of the Atlanta classification and definitions by international consensus. *Gut*. 2013;62:102.

Bassi C, Marchegiani G, Dervenis C, Sarr M, Abu Hilal M, et al. International Study Group on Pancreatic Surgery (ISGPS). The 2016 update of the International Study Group (ISGPS) definition and grading of postoperative pancreatic fistula: 11 years after. *Surgery*. 2017 Mar;161(3):584–591. doi: 10.1016/j.surg.2016.11.01D.

Bismuth H, Lazorthes F. Les *traumatismes operatoires de la voie biliare principale*. Paris, France: Masson, 1981.

Blumgart LH. *Surgery of the Liver, Biliary Tract and Pancreas*, 4th edition, Saunders, Philadelphia 2007.

Brunt LM, Deziel DJ, Telem DA, et al. Safe cholecystectomy multi-society practice guideline and state of the art consensus conference on prevention of bile duct injury during cholecystectomy. *Ann Surg*. 2020;272:3–23.

Chamberlain RS. *Hepatobiliary Surgery (Vademecum)*. 1st Edition, Kindle Edition by Author, 2003.

Chartrand-Lefebvre C, Dufresne M-P, Lafortune M, et al. Iatrogenic injury to the bile duct: A working classification for radiologists. *Radiology*. 1994;193:523.

Chen H, Siwo EA, Khu M, Tian Y. Current trends in the management of Mirizzi Syndrome: A review of literature. *Medicine (Baltimore)*. 2018 Jan;97(4):e9691. doi: 10.1097/MD.0000000000009691.

Crockett SD, Wani S, Gardner TB, et al. American Gastroenterological Association Institute Guideline on initial management of acute pancreatitis. *Gastroenterology*. 2018;154:1096.

Daamen LA, Dorland G, Brada LJH, Groot VP, van Oosten AF, Besselink MG et al. Dutch Pancreatic Cancer Group. Preoperative predictors for early and very early disease recurrence in patients undergoing resection of pancreatic ductal adenocarcinoma. *HPB (Oxford)*. 2021 Sep 24:S1365-182X(21)01624-5.

de Kleine RH, Schreuder AM, ten Hove A, et al. Choledochal malformations in adults in the Netherlands: results from a nationwide retrospective cohort study. *Liver Int*. 2020;40:2469.

Eshuis WJ, van er Gaag dNA, Rauws EA, van Eijck CH, Bruno MJ, Kuipers EJ, et al. Therapeutic delay and survival after surgery for cancer of the pancreatic head with or without preoperative biliary drainage. *Ann Surg*. 2010;252:840–849. doi: 10.1097/SLA.0b013e3181fd36a2.

Everhart JE, Ruhl CE. Burden of digestive diseases in the United States Part III: Liver, biliary tract, and pancreas. *Gastroenterology*. 2009;136:1134–1144.

Fang Y, Gurusamy KS, Wang Q, et al. Pre-operative biliary drainage for obstructive jaundice. *Cochrane Database Syst Rev*. 2012 Sep;12(9):CD005444

Fong Y, Jarnagin W, Blumgart LH. Gallbladder cancer: comparison of patients presenting initially for definitive operation with those presenting after prior noncurative intervention. *Ann Surg*. 2000;232:557.

Hartke J, Johnson M, Ghabril M. The diagnosis and treatment of hepatocellular carcinoma. *Semin Diagn Pathol*. 2017 Mar;34(2):153–159. doi: 10.1053/j.semdp.2016.12.011.

Heider TR, Azeem S, Galanko JA, Behrns KE. The natural history of pancreatitis-induced splenic vein thrombosis. *Ann Surg*. 2004;239:876.

Hess E, Thumbadoo RP, Thorne E, McNamee K. Gallstones in pregnancy. *Br J Hosp Med (Lond)*. 2021 Feb 2;82(2):1–8. doi: 10.12968/hmed.2020.0330.

Khatri VP, Petrelli NJ, Belghiti J. Extending the frontiers of surgical therapy for hepatic colorectal metastases: is there a limit? *J Clin Oncol*. 2005;23:8490.

Lahiri R, Bhattacharya S. Pancreatic trauma. *Ann R Coll Surg Engl*. 2013 May;95(4):241–5. doi: 10.1308/003588413X13629960045913.

Law R, Topazian M. Diagnosis and treatment of choledochoceles. *Clin Gastroenterol Hepatol*. 2014;12:196.

Marrero JA, Ahn J, Rajender Reddy K. American College of Gastroenterology. ACG clinical guideline: the diagnosis and management of focal liver lesions. *Am J Gastroenterol*. 2014 Sep;109(9):1328–1347; quiz 1348. doi: 10.1038/ajg.2014.213.

Massucco P, Capussotti L, Magnino A, et al. Pancreatic resections after chemoradiotherapy for locally advanced ductal adenocarcinoma: analysis of perioperative outcome and survival. *Ann Surg Oncol*. 2006;13:1201.

Mentha G, Majno PE, Andres A, et al. Neoadjuvant chemotherapy and resection of advanced synchronous liver metastases before treatment of the colorectal primary. *Br J Surg*. 2006;93:872.

National Comprehensive Cancer Network (NCCN). NCCN clinical practice guidelines in oncology. https://www.nccn.org/professionals/physician_gls (Accessed on November 09, 2021).

Norman Oneil Machado, Biliary complications post laparoscopic cholecystectomy: mechanism, preventive measures, and approach to management: a review. *Diagn Ther Endosc*. 2011;2011:Article ID 967017, 9 pages. doi:10.1155/2011/967017.

Padillo FJ, Andicoberry B, Naranjoet A, et al. Anorexia and the effect of internal biliary drainage on food intake in patients with obstructive jaundice. *J Am Coll Surg*. 2001 May;192(5):584–590

Pawlik TM, Gleisner AL, Vigano L, et al. Incidence of finding residual disease for incidental gallbladder carcinoma: implications for re-resection. *J Gastrointest Surg*. 2007;11:1478.

Rahnemai-Azar AA, Selby LV, Lustberg MB, Pawlik TM. Surgical management of breast cancer liver metastasis. *Surg Oncol Clin N Am*. 2021 Jan;30(1):27–37. doi: 10.1016/j. soc.2020.09.003.

Ribero D, Pinna AD, Guglielmi A, et al. Surgical approach for long-term survival of patients with intrahepatic cholangiocarcinoma: a multi-institutional analysis of 434 patients. *Arch Surg*. 2012;147(12):1107–1113. doi:10.1001/archsurg.2012.1962.

Sanford DE. An update on technical aspects of cholecystectomy. *Surg Clin North Am*. 2019 Apr;99(2):245–258. doi: 10.1016/j.suc.2018.11.005.

Scheiman JM, Hwang JH, Moayyedi P. American Gastroenterological Association technical review on the diagnosis and management of asymptomatic neoplastic pancreatic cysts. *Gastroenterology*. 2015 Apr;148(4):824–48.e22. doi: 10.1053/j. gastro.2015.01.014.

Schulick RD. Criteria of unresectability and the decision-making process. *HPB (Oxford)*. 2008;10(2):122–125. doi:10.1080/13651820801993540.

Seufferlein T, Bachet JB, Van Cutsem E, et al. Pancreatic adenocarcinoma: ESMO-ESDO Clinical Practice Guidelines for diagnosis, treatment and follow-up. *Ann Oncol*. 2012;23 Suppl 7:vii33.

Sharma A, Sharma KL, Gupta A, et al. Gallbladder cancer epidemiology, pathogenesis and molecular genetics: recent update. *World J Gastroenterol*. 2017;23:3978.

Shen Z, Zhang J, Zhao S, et al. Preoperative biliary drainage of severely obstructive jaundiced patients decreases overall postoperative complications after pancreaticoduodenectomy: a retrospective and propensity score-matched analysis. *Pancreatology*. 2020 Apr;20(3):529–536.

Singham J, Yoshida EM, Scudamore CH. Choledochal cysts. Part 3 of 3: management. *Can J Surg*. 2010;53:51.

Slesser AA, Simillis C, Goldin R, et al. A meta-analysis comparing simultaneous versus delayed resections in patients with synchronous colorectal liver metastases. *Surg Oncol*. 2013;22:36.

Søreide K, Søreide JA. Bile duct cyst as precursor to biliary tract cancer. *Ann Surg Oncol*. 2007;14:1200.

Strasberg SM, Brunt LM. Rationale and use of the critical view of safety in laparoscopic cholecystectomy. *J Am Coll Surg*. 2010;211:132–138.

Strasberg SM, Hertl M, Soper NJ. An analysis of the problem of biliary injury during laparoscopic cholecystectomy. *J Am Coll Surg*. 1995;180:101.

Suzuki M, Akaishi S, Rikiyama T, Naitoh T, Rahman MM, Matsuno S. Laparoscopic cholecystectomy, Calot's triangle, and variations in cystic arterial supply. *Surg Endosc*. 2000 Feb;14(2):141–144.

Tanaka M, Chari S, Adsay V, Fernandez-del Castillo C, Falconi M, Shimizu M, Yamaguchi K, Yamao K, Matsuno S. International Association of Pancreatology. International consensus guidelines for management of intraductal papillary mucinous neoplasms and mucinous cystic neoplasms of the pancreas. *Pancreatology*. 2006;6(1–2):17–32. doi: 10.1159/000090023.

Todani T, Watanabe Y, Narusue M, Tabuchi K, Okajima K. Congenital bile duct cysts. Classification, operative procedures, and review of thirty-seven cases including cancer arising from choledochal cyst. *Am J Surg*. 1977;134(2):263–269.

van Baal MC, Bollen TL, Bakker OJ, van Goor H, Boermeester MA, Dejong CH, Gooszen HG, van der Harst E, van Eijck CH, van Santvoort HC, Besselink MG; Dutch Pancreatitis Study Group. The role of routine fine-needle aspiration in the diagnosis of infected necrotizing pancreatitis. *Surgery*. 2014 Mar;155(3):442–448. doi: 10.1016/j. surg.2013.10.001.

van Brunschot S, van Grinsven J, van Santvoort HC, Bakker OJ, Besselink MG, Boermeester MA, Bollen TL, Bosscha K, Bouwense SA, Bruno MJ, Cappendijk VC, Consten EC, Dejong CH, van Eijck CH, Erkelens WG, van Goor H, van Grevenstein WMU, Haveman JW, Hofker SH, Jansen JM, Laméris JS, van Lienden KP, Meijssen MA, Mulder CJ, Nieuwenhuijs VB, Poley JW, Quispel R, de Ridder RJ, Römkens TE, Scheepers JJ, Schepers NJ, Schwartz MP, Seerden T, Spanier BWM, Straathof JWA, Strijker M, Timmer R, Venneman NG, Vleggaar FP, Voermans RP, Witteman BJ, Gooszen HG, Dijkgraaf MG, Fockens P; Dutch Pancreatitis Study Group. Endoscopic or surgical step-up approach for infected necrotising pancreatitis: a multicentre randomised trial. *Lancet*. 2018 Jan 6;391(10115):51–58. doi: 10.1016/ S0140-6736(17)32404-2.

Van Der Gaag NA, Kloek JJ, De Castro SM, et al. Preoperative biliary drainage in patients with obstructive jaundice: history and current status. *J Gastrointest Surg*. 2009 Apr;13(4):814–820.

van Grinsven J, van Dijk SM, Dijkgraaf MG, Boermeester MA, Bollen TL, Bruno MJ, van Brunschot S, Dejong CH, van Eijck CH, van Lienden KP, Boerma D, van Duijvendijk P, Hadithi M, Haveman JW, van der Hulst RW, Jansen JM, Lips DJ, Manusama ER, Molenaar IQ, van der Peet DL, Poen AC, Quispel R, Schaapherder AF, Schoon EJ, Schwartz MP, Seerden TC, Spanier BWM, Straathof JW, Venneman NG, van de Vrie W, Witteman BJ, van Goor H, Fockens P, van Santvoort HC, Besselink MG; Dutch

Pancreatitis Study Group. Postponed or immediate drainage of infected necrotizing pancreatitis (POINTER trial): study protocol for a randomized controlled trial. *Trials.* 2019 Apr 25;20(1):239. doi: 10.1186/s13063-019-3315-6.

Van Santvoort HC, Besselink MG, Cirkel GA, Gooszen HG. Landelijk onderzoek naar optimale behandeling van patiënten met geïnfecteerde necrotiserende pancreatitis: PANTER-trial [A nationwide Dutch study into the optimal treatment of patients with infected necrotising pancreatitis: the PANTER trial]. *Ned Tijdschr Geneeskd.* 2006 Aug 19;150(33):1844–1846.

Weyant MJ, Maluccio MA, Bertagnolli MM, Daly JM. Choledochal cysts in adults: a report of two cases and review of the literature. *Am J Gastroenterol.* 1998;93:2580.

Wolfe D, Kanji S, Yazdi F, Barbeau P, Rice D, Beck A, Butler C, Esmaeilisaraji L, Skidmore B, Moher D, Hutton B. Drug induced pancreatitis: a systematic review of case reports to determine potential drug associations. *PLoS One.* 2020 Apr 17;15(4):e0231883. doi: 10.1371/journal.pone.0231883.

Working Group IAP/APA Acute Pancreatitis Guidelines. IAP/APA evidence-based guidelines for the management of acute pancreatitis. *Pancreatology.* 2013;13:e1.

Zhou MT, Chen CS, Chen BC, Zhang QY, Andersson R. Acute lung injury and ARDS in acute pancreatitis: mechanisms and potential intervention. *World J Gastroenterol.* 2010 May 7;16(17):2094–9. doi: 10.3748/wjg.v16.i17.2094.

7 Oesophagogastric Surgery

Yuen Soon and Tanvir Hossain

Q1. A 56-year-old man has a gastrooesophageal junctional tumour that appears to originate in the proximal stomach 3 cm distal to the GOJ and extends up towards the GOJ. What Siewert classification is this?
  A. Siewert type 1
  B. Siewert type 2
  C. Siewert type 3
  D. Siewert type 4
  E. Siewert type 5

Q2. A 39-year-old man has been binge-drinking over the course of the day following the FA cup final. He eats a large donner kebab very quickly after all the bars have closed and his last bite of the kebab in his taxi home was followed by violent vomiting. He presents to the emergency department 4 hours later septic with severe chest pain. ECG shows sinus tachycardia. How would you manage this patient?
  A. Endosponge
  B. Chest drain, NBM, OGD and nasojejunal tube
  C. Right side thoracotomy, washout and Ivor-Lewis oesophagectomy
  D. On-table gastroscopy, left thoracotomy, washout, insertion of drains and t-tube followed by laparotomy and feeding jejunostomy
  E. Chest drain only

Q3. Which is the most common *Helicobacter pylori*-associated lymphoma?
  A. T-cell lymphoma
  B. MALToma
  C. Nodular sclerosing Hodgkin's lymphoma
  D. Mixed cellularity Hodgkin's lymphoma
  E. Lymphocyte-depleted lymphoma

Q4. Resection of which of the following does not require lymphadenectomy?
  A. Sigmoid cancer
  B. GIST of the stomach
  C. Intestinal carcinoid
  D. Lower oesophageal adenocarcinoma
  E. Head of the pancreas adenocarcinoma

DOI: 10.1201/9781003221234-7

Q5. Which is true regarding the blood supply of the stomach?
   A. The right gastroepiploic is a branch of the common hepatic artery
   B. The right gastric artery is a branch of the gastroduodenal artery
   C. The left gastroepiploic artery is a branch of the splenic artery
   D. The short gastric arteries supply the distal stomach
   E. The left gastric artery is a branch of the superior mesenteric artery

Q6. Which of the following is not a pathological feature of a GIST which can aid histological diagnosis?
   A. Stipple cells
   B. CD34
   C. CD117
   D. Spindle cells
   E. DOG1

Q7. A 64-year-old man with COPD and IHD has a 3 cm adenocarcinoma in the body of the stomach. What are the surgical options?
   A. Wide local excision with a 2 cm margin
   B. Total gastrectomy and lymphadenectomy
   C. Total gastrectomy with oesophagojejunostomy and Roux-en-Y reconstruction with feeding jejunostomy
   D. Subtotal gastrectomy
   E. Wide local excision with 1 cm margin

Q8. During a laparoscopic fundoplication, what are the life-threatening complications that can arise
   A. Lung injury
   B. Massive haemorrhage
   C. Cardiac tamponade
   D. Air embolism
   E. Saddle embolus

Q9. What is the surveillance modality after an Ivor-Lewis oesophagectomy for a T3N1 M0 tumour of the lower oesophagus?
   A. Annual CT for 5 years, OGD at 1 year, and tumour markers every 3 months for 5 years
   B. Gastroscopy at 1 year, then yearly until year 5
   C. Clinical follow-up alone
   D. CT 6, 18, 24 months then years 3, 4, 5
   E. MRI liver years 2, 3 and 5

Q10. In patients with iron deficiency anaemia when undergoing gastroscopy
   A. D2 biopsies should be performed
   B. Antral biopsies are required to exclude gastritis as a cause of bleeding
   C. Antral biopsies are required to exclude *H. pylori* as the cause for gastritis causing bleeding
   D. CLO test should be performed to exclude *H. pylori*
   E. No mandatory biopsies but lesions should be biopsied

Q11. A patient is diagnosed clinically with 2 cm of circumferential columnar-lined oesophagus. Biopsies confirm columnar mucosa, but no features of intestinal metaplasia are identified. What is the most appropriate follow-up for this patient?

    A. Repeat OGD in 6 weeks after treatment with PPI
    B. Surveillance endoscopy in 1 year
    C. Repeat endoscopy in 3 years
    D. No surveillance
    E. Surveillance endoscopy in 3–5 years of surgery

Q12. Which of the following is false regarding *H. pylori*?

    A. Approximately 95% of duodenal ulcers that are not caused by NSAIDs are associated with *H. pylori*
    B. It causes a chronic inflammatory process in the stomach causing gastric atrophy
    C. It is a Gram-positive helical-shaped bacillus
    D. *H. Pylori* is associated with an increased risk of gastric adenocarcinoma
    E. Produces urease

Q13. A 38-year-old man with 10 pack-year smoking history and 80 U/week ETOH intake presents with peritonitis and was found to have a 1 cm perforation at the gastric antrum. How will you manage this?

    A. Distal gastrectomy
    B. Biopsy and T-Tube
    C. Primary closure
    D. Biopsy and omental patch
    E. Duodenal exclusion and gastrojejunostomy

Q14. A 57-year-old man with lower oesophageal cancer is undergoing staging. He has dysphagia to solids and has lost 16 kg in weight. At gastroscopy, the tumour is narrowing the lumen, but the scope is able to pass it. How will you address the nutritional challenge?

    A. Stent at OGD
    B. Stent + feeding jejunostomy
    C. TPN
    D. Nutrition team referral and consideration for prescription of liquid diet
    E. Nasojejunal feeding tube

Q15. A 63-year-old lady awaiting total knee replacement presents with upper GI perforation. A 3 cm perforation of the D1 ulcer is found at laparoscopy. Select the most appropriate management.

    A. Duodenal exclusion and gastrojejunostomy
    B. Primary closure
    C. Omental patch alone
    D. Distal gastrectomy
    E. Close over a foley catheter

Q16. Which of the following do NOT require D2 biopsies at gastroscopy?
   A. Niacin deficiency
   B. Iron deficiency anaemia
   C. Folate deficiency
   D. IgA endomysial antibodies
   E. Osteomalacia

Q17. A patient is diagnosed clinically with 2 cm of circumferential Barrett's oesophagus. What is the minimum number of biopsies that should be taken?
   A. 1
   B. 2
   C. 4
   D. 8
   E. 10

Q18. A 28-year-old patient had an endoscopic insertion of a PEG. That evening the patient has abdominal pain and tachycardia with a heart rate of 100. The patient has a tender epigastrium however arterial blood gas result is normal. What is your next step?
   A. Manage with analgesia and observe
   B. Erect CXR
   C. CT with IV and PEG contrast
   D. CT with IV and oral contrast
   E. Gastrograffin via PEG with imaging in the fluoroscopy department

Q19. A 52-year-old man with no comorbidities has HGD noted on Barret's oesophagus biopsies, he undergoes EMR with R0 resection. Subsequent surveillance shows a further lesion, and piecemeal biopsy shows adenocarcinoma, its piecemeal nature deemed the report as R1. What surgical opinion do you give at the MDT?
   A. Oesophagectomy
   B. Observe and re-scope ± further EMR
   C. Radiofrequency ablation
   D. Neoadjuvant chemotherapy
   E. Radiotherapy

Q20. A 73-year-old man has suspected gastric cancer through gastroscopy. The patient was on clopidogrel for a PCI stent performed in the previous year. How do you proceed?
   A. Ask the patient to stop clopidogrel and return in 7 days
   B. Ask the patient to stop clopidogrel and return in 14 days
   C. Give vitamin K and proceed to biopsy
   D. Give TXA and proceed to biopsy
   E. Take the biopsy

Q21. A 32-year patient old man undergoes a Nissen's fundoplication for pathological reflux confirmed on pH studies, he has normal motility. He calls the team 4 weeks after the operation complaining of frequent diarrhoea. What is the likely cause?
A. C. difficile
B. Vagus nerve damage
C. Continued need for a liquid diet
D. Overtight wrap
E. Coeliacs disease

Q22. A 64-year-old man at gastroscopy is found to have a Siewert type 1 GOJ. Following this, the patient presents to the emergency department with tachycardia, pyrexia and surgical emphysema. A CT chest/abdomen diagnoses a perforated T3 tumour. What is the best management option?
A. Laparoscopic feeding jejunostomy and endoscopic insertion of an uncovered stent
B. Emergency extended total gastrectomy
C. Conservative management with keeping NBM, IV antibiotics
D. Emergency Ivor-Lewis oesophagectomy
E. Endoscopic insertion of a fully covered stent

Q23. A 41-year-old lady with dyspepsia undergoes a gastroscopy where hyperplastic polyps are found. The trainee endoscopist was unsure of what to do next and discusses with you the management. What do you advise?
A. Reassure no further action is required
B. Start triple therapy
C. Test for *H. pylori* and follow-up in 12 months
D. Test for *H. pylori* and follow-up OGD in 3 years
E. Annual surveillance for 5 years

Q24. An optimal site for open chest drain insertion on the left side is?
A. Midaxillary point in the seventh intercostal space
B. Midclavicular line fifth intercostal space
C. Anywhere in the fifth intercostal space where there is the least soft tissue to cross
D. Midaxillary line fifth intercostal space
E. Second intercostal space, mid axillary line

Q25. A 59-year-old man has undergone an OGD, CT chest/abdomen, PET CT scan and staging laparoscopy diagnosing T3N1M0 adenocarcinoma of the distal oesophagus not involving GOJ. What is the next management step for this patient?
A. Direct to surgery
B. Neoadjuvant chemotherapy
C. Surgery with adjuvant radiotherapy
D. EMR
E. Chemoradiotherapy

Q26. A 52-year-old lady who lives alone is being investigated for chronic anaemia on the day of the gastroscopy mentions she is also beginning to get dysphagia to some solids. What is the diagnosis?
   A.   Haemorrhagic gastritis
   B.   Gastric cancer
   C.   Achalasia
   D.   Jack Hammer syndrome
   E.   Plummer–Vinson syndrome

Q27. Which of the following is true of gastric cancer?
   A.   Intestinal type has an equal male: female distribution
   B.   Diffuse type has an association with atrophic gastritis
   C.   Intestinal type occurs in an older population than the diffuse type
   D.   Adenocarcinomas make up 50% of gastric cancers
   E.   Intestinal-type gastric cancers have signet rings

Q28. A 48-year-old lady had a 4 cm GIST with a low mitotic count resected by open distal gastrectomy. She presents 18 months later with lower abdominal pain and a CT scan shows a recurrence in the pelvis. How should this be managed?
   A.   Radiotherapy
   B.   Radical resection with pelvic exenteration
   C.   Tyrosine kinase inhibitor
   D.   Limited resection and tyrosine kinase inhibitor
   E.   Chemotherapy

Q29. The following characteristics are not appropriate for the endoscopic management of gastric cancer?
   A.   No disease
   B.   A non-ulcerated lesion
   C.   T1a/T1b tumour
   D.   Well-differentiated lesion
   E.   Lesions 2 cm in size

Q30. A 47-year-old man who had a GIST resected in 2019 has represented a recurrence involving multiple sites in the abdomen. The original resected tumour was 5 cm in size and was described as a wild-type GIST. What is the management?
   A.   Straight to surgery
   B.   Downstage with imatinib and re-scan with the view to operating
   C.   Palliative care
   D.   Radiotherapy
   E.   Sunitinib

Q31. A 64-year-old smoker presents with dyspepsia, dysphagia to some solids and 6 kg weight loss over 2 months. A barium swallow report described a rat's tail appearance. What is the likely diagnosis?
   A.   Arterial lusoria
   B.   Oesophageal cancer
   C.   Benign oesophageal stricture
   D.   Type 2 achalasia
   E.   Scleroderma

Q32. A 63-year-old man undergoes a gastroscopy and is found to have a stricture which cannot be passed. You are unable to get adequate biopsies. How do you proceed?
  A. Balloon dilatation of the lesion and then take four biopsies from within the lesion
  B. Dilate using a Savary-Gilliard dilator and then two biopsies
  C. Switch to the paediatric scope and attempt six biopsies
  D. Abandon and request radiologically guided biopsy
  E. Abandon the procedure and discuss it in MDT

Q33. A depressed colorectal surgeon presents to the emergency department 3 hours after swallowing 300 mL of bleach. What is the next step?
  A. Emergency laparotomy and right hemicolectomy
  B. Clinical observation and keep nil by mouth
  C. Urgent gastroscopy
  D. Next day gastroscopy
  E. Three-stage oesophagectomy

Q34. Of the following assessment/investigations, which is not mandatory before performing anti-reflux surgery?
  A. 24-hour pH studies
  B. Manometry studies
  C. Clinical assessment
  D. OGD
  E. Flexible sigmoidoscopy

Q35. A 68-year-old lady undergoes a gastroscopy for dyspepsia and water brash. After a few attempts, the oesophagus is intubated and entered and the test is performed with a 3 cm hiatus hernia, but nothing else is noted. The patient returns to the hospital the next day with chest pain and surgical emphysema in the neck. The patient is otherwise well, not septic and haemodynamically stable. A CT with oral contrast shows a perforation at the level of the neck. How should this be managed?
  A. Three-stage oesophagectomy
  B. Open surgery with the stapled repair of the diverticulum
  C. Endoscopy and clipping of perforation
  D. OGD and insertion of the nasojejunal feeding tube
  E. Keep NBM and TPN

Q36. A 47-year-old lady with no paraoesophageal hernia and no other comorbidities presents to the emergency department with vomiting, upper abdominal pain for 6 hours, tachycardia, and hypotension and has haematemesis of approx. 300 mL. The CT scanner is out of order. What is your management strategy?
  A. Refer to medics, obtain Rockall score and admit to gastroenterology for urgent gastroscopy
  B. Stabilise patient with fluids IV antibiotics and request an urgent USS of the abdomen
  C. Book for an emergency theatre for laparotomy and on-table gastroscopy
  D. Give vitamin K, blood transfusion and admit for observation in the surgical ward
  E. Book an elective fundoplication

Q37. A 78-year-old man with worsening dysphagia has a barium swallow. This shows a fixed narrowing of the upper oesophagus. What is your next step?

A. Gastroscopy

B. pH/Manometry studies

C. Bravo

D. POEM

E. Cardiomyotomy

Q38. A 74-year-old patient with a BMI of 40 and poor mobility undergoes an Ivor-Lewis oesophagectomy. He spikes a temperature of 38.1 degrees on the fifth postoperative day. He has a CT with oral contrast which does not show any extravasation of contrast from the anastomosis but does note bilateral chest atelectasis and is commenced on IV antibiotics for LRTI. What is the most effective strategy to prevent this?

A. Prehabilitation programme

B. Pre-operative chlorhexidine mouthwashes

C. Protective ventilation and thoracic epidural analgesia

D. Daily bronchoscopy and washout

E. Partnership programme with geriatrician for post-op reviews

Q39. A 52-year-old man presents with haematemesis, emergency gastroscopy shows a bleeding vessel that is injected with adrenaline. The bleeding significantly reduces. What is your next step?

A. Admit and re-scope in 24 hours

B. Discharge

C. Give 1 g TXA and admit for further two doses over 24 hours

D. Clip the vessel

E. Book CT angio ± embolisation

Q40. A 43-year-old alcoholic presented with upper GI perforation and has a patch repair of a perforated duodenal ulcer. He is prescribed triple therapy and discharged on a postoperative day 3. Select the correct one. What is the next step?

A. Chase histology report

B. Serum IgG levels should be scheduled to confirm eradication

C. His *H. pylori* status should be checked with a C13/14 breath test in 8 to confirm *H. pylori* eradication

D. Book gastroscopy to ensure healing of the ulcer and CLO test

E. No further action

Q41. A 56-year-old lady presented with an epigastric mass. CT of the abdomen shows a 10 cm gastric GIST involving the body of the pancreas. Subsequent EUS confirms this. What is the next step?

A. Resect GIST en bloc with distal pancreatectomy and splenectomy

B. Downstage with imatinib

C. Conservative management

D. Resect GIST off the pancreas

E. Palliation

Q42. A 32-year-old lady with dysphagia is found to have type 2 achalasia. What is the most appropriate treatment option?
   A. Balloon dilatation
   B. POEM
   C. Dor fundoplication
   D. Laparoscopic cardiomyotomy with gastropexy
   E. Botulinum injection

Q43. For a 67-year-old man with a lower oesophageal adenocarcinoma staged T1N0M0, what appropriate management would be?
   A. Ivor-Lewis oesophagectomy
   B. Transhiatal oesophagectomy
   C. Chemoradiotherapy
   D. EMR
   E. Neoadjuvant chemotherapy

Q44. A 70-year-old man has an Ivor-Lewis oesophagectomy. He presents with massive hematemesis on day 1 post-op. A gastroscopy shows a stomach full of blood. Endoscopic management fails and he is haemodynamically unstable. He undergoes an angiogram and coiling of the gastroduodenal artery. What are your concerns?
   A. Thromboembolism
   B. Re-bleeding
   C. Massive MI
   D. CVA
   E. Ischaemic gastric conduit

Q45. Which of the following is NOT true of feeding nasogastric tubes?
   A. NG tubes do not need for X-ray for checking the position
   B. 10–12F tubes are optimal for feeding
   C. Long-term NG tubes should be changed every 6 weeks
   D. NG tube insertion should be avoided for 3 days in the event of an acute variceal bleeding
   E. pH testing is required for checking the position of feeding NG tubes

Q46. A 52-year-old man presents with haematemesis and undergoes gastroscopy. An ulcer is found at D1 that has failed endoscopic therapy. Interventional radiology performs angioembolisation and this fail. What is the next step?
   A. Repeat endoscopic attempt as embolisation would make success more likely
   B. Repeat angioembolisation
   C. Liaise with haematology and request prothrombin complex concentrate
   D. Perform distal gastrectomy
   E. Laparotomy and underrunning of ulcer

Q47. A 49-year-old man has been found to have a GOJ adenocarcinoma. A CT of the chest/abdomen/pelvis and PET CT have not noted any metastatic disease. EUS has confirmed no local metastases and a T2 tumour. What is the next step?
   A. Neoadjuvant chemotherapy
   B. Radiotherapy
   C. Straight to surgery
   D. Oesophageal stent (uncovered)
   E. Staging laparoscopy

Q48. You are unable to pass D2 at gastroscopy for a patient that has presented with abdominal distention and vomiting. It is collapsed, although the mucosa appears normal. What is the cause?
   A. Duodenal ulcer
   B. Duodenal cancer
   C. Adhesions
   D. Extrinsic compression
   E. Gastric ulcer

Q49. A gentleman with long-term progressive dysphagia; endoscopy is normal; barium swallow shows fixed narrowing of the upper oesophagus.
   A. Leiomyoma
   B. Achalasia
   C. Cardiospasm
   D. Zenker's diverticulum
   E. Dysphagia lusoria

Q50. What is the best indication for a satisfactory response from anti-reflux surgery in pathological reflux?
   A. Demeester score
   B. Response to PPI
   C. Symptomatic relief
   D. Age
   E. Previous surgery

Q51. A 48-year-old lady with Barrett's oesophagus had biopsies confirming high-grade dysplasia. What are the circumstances in which HGS is confirmed?
   A. At least two concurrent episodes of HGD on biopsies are required therefore book a repeat gastroscopy and biopsy
   B. High clinical suspicion
   C. Pathologist confirmation
   D. Two Pathologists have to confirm
   E. Only in known Barrett's cases

Q52. The following conditions do not predispose to oesophageal cancer
   A. Achalasia
   B. Plummer–Vinson Syndrome
   C. Obesity
   D. Reflux
   E. Carney Syndrome

Q53. The following has the least association with gastric cancer
   A. *Helicobacter pylori*
   B. Alcohol
   C. Reflux
   D. Lynch Syndrome
   E. FAP

Q54. Neuroendocrine tumours of the stomach:
   A. Type 1 tumours are usually single and found in men
   B. In type 2 tumours, Ki67 is usually >2
   C. In type 1 tumours, there is never any risk of metastases
   D. In type 3 tumours, one-third have died in 51 months
   E. In type 3 tumours, the patient usually presents with multiple polypoidal tumours

Q55. The following are not criteria for screening of hereditary diffuse gastric cancer
   A. Three or more cases of gastric cancer in the family
   B. Individual with lobular breast cancer and diffuse gastric cancer
   C. Isolated individual with diffuse gastric cancer under 40
   D. Family history of ductal breast cancer and diffuse gastric cancer
   E. Family history of signet ring colon cancer and diffuse gastric cancer

Q56. Staging, the following are not routine staging modalities for gastric cancer
   A. OGD
   B. Biopsy
   C. CT scan
   D. PET scan
   E. Laparoscopy

Q57. Treatment of junctional gastrooesophageal cancer
   A. The treatment is always neoadjuvant chemotherapy followed by surgery
   B. The treatment is always surgery first
   C. The treatment must always include chemotherapy
   D. The treatment is best with radiotherapy
   E. The treatment must be discussed in a multidisciplinary team

Q58. In gastric cancer with only peritoneal disease in an otherwise fit patient keen on curative therapy, the treatment modalities are:
   A. Intraperitoneal chemotherapy
   B. Radical surgery
   C. Systemic chemotherapy
   D. Best supportive care
   E. Radiotherapy

Q59. All junctional cancers must be treated
   A. By two-phase oesophagogastrectomy
   B. By three-phase oesophagogastrectomy
   C. By total gastrectomy
   D. By proximal gastrectomy
   E. Be discussed in a multidisciplinary team

Q60. Minimally invasive oesophagectomy
    A. Has lower 30-day mortality
    B. Has higher 30-day mortality
    C. Has a lower readmission rate
    D. Has a higher reoperation rate
    E. Has a lower reoperation rate

Q61. Minimally invasive oesophagectomy with cervical anastomosis when compared
    to intrathoracic anastomosis in minimally invasive oesophagectomy
    A. Has a higher severe complication rate
    B. Has a lower severe complication rate
    C. Shorter ITU stay
    D. Longer ITU stay
    E. Lower mortality

Q62. In an oesophagectomy for distal oesophageal cancer, the aim of surgery includes
    A. Removal of primary tumour only
    B. Removal of the primary tumour with one-phase lymphadenectomy
    C. Removal of the primary tumour with two-phase lymphadenectomy
    D. Removal of the primary tumour with three-phase lymphadenectomy
    E. Removal of the primary tumour with four-phase lymphadenectomy

Q63. Palliative management of gastric cancer does not include
    A. Chemotherapy
    B. Total gastrectomy
    C. Gastric bypass
    D. Stent
    E. Radiotherapy

Q64. Reflux is unlikely to be associated with
    A. Globus
    B. Asthma
    C. Otitis media
    D. Progressive dysphagia
    E. Cough

Q65. In a young patient with persistent reflux symptoms despite maximal PPI therapy,
    the following is indicated:
    A. Barium swallow
    B. pH impedance manometry on PPI
    C. CT scan of the abdomen
    D. Electrogastrogram
    E. Increase PPI treatment to BD dosing

Q66. The half-life of omeprazole is
    A. 48 hours
    B. 24 hours
    C. 12 hours
    D. 6 hours
    E. Under 3 hours

Q67. The following medications require acid to activate it
  A. H2 antagonist
  B. Magnesium trisilicate
  C. Aluminium hydroxide
  D. Sucralfate
  E. PPI

Q68. The following are not mechanisms of oesophageal continence
  A. Intra-abdominal oesopagus
  B. Angle of His
  C. Lower oesophageal sphincter
  D. Diaphragmatic sphincter
  E. Raised intra-abdominal pressure

Q69. Hiatus hernias usually present
  A. Present with epigastric tenderness
  B. Shortness of breast
  C. Epigastric pain
  D. Coughing
  E. Asymptomatically

Q70. In hiatal hernia repair, the aims of surgery do not include
  A. Reduction of hernia
  B. Excision of the hernia sac
  C. Reduction of 2–3 cm of the oesophagus to the abdomen
  D. Repair of the crus with a mesh
  E. Fundoplication

Q71. Studies show that Toupet's fundoplication vs Nissen's fundoplication
  A. Toupet is better at preventing reflux than Nissen
  B. Nissen is better at preventing reflux than Toupet
  C. Toupet has a better air swallowing side effect profile than Nissen
  D. Nissen has a better air swallowing side effect profile than Toupet
  E. Nissen last longer than Toupet fundoplication

Q72. Achalasia is defined by
  A. Abnormal IRP and normal peristalsis
  B. Normal IRP and normal peristalsis
  C. Abnormal IRP and abnormal peristalsis
  D. Abnormal IRP and absent peristalsis
  E. Normal IRP and absent peristalsis

Q73. Primary management of type 2 achalasia in a young patient with grade 1–3 oesophageal dilatation does not include:
  A. Stapled cardioplasty
  B. Botox injection into the GEJ
  C. POEM
  D. Laparoscopic Heller myotomy
  E. Pneumatic dilatation

Q74. Counselling patients with achalasia, the major difference in POEM vs laparoscopic Hellers cardiomyotomy is:
A. Postoperative dysphagia
B. Postoperative hospital stay
C. Postoperative morbidity and mortality
D. Postoperative reflux
E. Postoperative scarring

Q75. Persistent dysphagia post-myotomy must be investigated by
A. pH manometry
B. Endoscopy
C. Barium swallow
D. CT scan
E. PET scan

ANSWERS

Q1. Option C – Siewert type 3.
A Siewert type 1 tumour originates >1 cm proximal to the GOJ, a type 2 between 1 cm proximal to the GOJ and 2 cm distal to the GOJ - a true tumour of the cardia. A type 3 tumour infiltrates the GOJ from more than 2 cm distal to the GOJ.

Q2. Option D – On-table gastroscopy, left thoracotomy, washout, insertion of drains and t-tube followed by laparotomy and feeding jejunostomy.
The management of Boerharve's depends on contamination, stability and fitness of the patient. All-day drinking and a full-size kebab may not be amenable to endosponge if there is significant contamination and mediastinitis. Perforations are usually on the left side; however, table gastroscopy is good practice prior to surgery. There is an alternative view for avoiding the laparotomy if contamination is all in the chest and inserting a nasojejunal tube instead; however, these can block or fall out.

Q3. Option B – MALToma.
Mucosa-associated lymphoid tissue lymphoma (MALToma) is the most common *H. pylori*-associated lymphoma. *H. pylori* eradication is the preferred treatment as the tumour may regress on treatment.

Q4. Option B – GIST of the stomach.
GIST is unlikely to have lymphatic spread

Q5. Option C – The left gastroepiploic artery is a branch of the splenic artery.
The stomach's predominant blood supply is from the left gastric artery, a branch from the coeliac trunk it is usually taken with cancer resections. The right gastric artery branches from the common hepatic artery. The right gastroepiploic is vital if using the distal stomach as a conduit and branches from the gastroduodenal artery. The left gastroepiploic artery branches, like the short gastric from the splenic artery and this complex, is vital for the remanent pouch in a subtotal or distal gastrectomy.

Q6. Option A – Stipple cells.

GISTs are often spindle cell tumours that arise in the smooth muscle pacemaker interstitial cell of Cajal and are driven by mutations in the KIT, PDGFRA or BRAF kinase genes. Most stain for KIT (CD117) and CD34. DOG1 antibody is sensitive and specific to GISTS in cytology cell blocks. Stipple cells are blood cells containing basophilic-staining bodies.

Q7. Option D – Subtotal gastrectomy.

If a stomach pouch is feasible after the resection of cancer with appropriate margins it has a better functional outcome than a total gastrectomy.

Q8. Option C – Cardiac tamponade.

Q9. Option C – Clinical follow-up alone.

Recurrence of the disease would not lead to further resection as there would be no survival benefit. Therefore clinical follow-up alone is done.

Q10. Option A – D2 biopsies should be performed.

D2 biopsies are required to exclude coeliac disease. The best practice is for D2 biopsy only after a positive serological test for anti-tissue transglutaminase antibody (tTG) or a negative test with a high clinical suspicion as per BSG guidelines.

Q11. Option D – No surveillance.

Q12. Option C – t is a gram-positive helical-shaped bacillus.

H. Pylori is a gram-negative microaerophilic helical-shaped bacillus.

Q13. Option D – Biopsy and omental patch.

Gastric ulcers should have samples taken for histological analysis. Primary repair±omental patch repairs are acceptable depending on the size of the ulcer.

Q14. Option E – Nasojejunal feeding tube.

There are a number of approaches to this problem, in general, enteral routes for feeding are preferred and they can be done in the community. A stent as a bridge to surgery is discouraged by a number of studies and guidelines but is practised in some centres. The ability to tolerate liquids means an oral liquid diet is feasible; however, the significant weight loss means NJ feed is preferred.

Q15. Option D – Distal gastrectomy.

This size perforation would be difficult to close primarily, with the risk of narrowing the duodenum. A distal gastrectomy would be the best approach here with a drain, should there be a duodenal stump leak.

Q16. Option E – Osteomalacia.

Patients with suspected coeliac disease and a positive TTG (or negative TTG yet still high suspicion of coeliac disease) should have a D2 biopsy. These would be patients with iron deficiency, folate deficiency, osteomalacia, or weight loss. IgA endomysial antibodies patients should not avoid eating gluten prior to the biopsy such that villous atrophy and intraepithelial lymphocytosis that is characteristic of coeliacs can be identified.

Q17. Option C – 4.

Four quadrant biopsies should be taken every 2 cm

Q18. Option D – CT with iv and oral contrast.

The concern would be for complications including damage to the colon as well as leakage from the peg.

Q19. Option A – Oesophagectomy.

This is a challenging discussion with the patient; theoretically, the piecemeal biopsy could have completely excised cancer, in a fit patient ILO would be the safest option, in unfit patient surveillance ±, further EMR is a possibility

Q20. Option E – Take the biopsy.

This is a low-risk intervention in a low risk for thromboembolic event patients.

Q21. Option B – Vagus nerve damage.

The diarrhoea may be because of damage to the Vagus nerve during the operation.

Q22. Option D – Emergency Ivor-Lewis oesophagectomy.

Conservative options may settle the patient's symptoms but a definitive procedure for those who are fit is better in a perforated oesophageal tumour.

Q23. Option C – Test for *H. pylori* and follow up in 12 months.

Hyperplastic polyps are often *H. pylori*-associated; thus, testing is recommended by the BSG guidelines. There is no evidence of benefit from long-term surveillance; however, there is a small (2%) associated cancer risk; therefore, a 12-month follow-up is recommended.

Q24. Option D – Midaxillary line fifth intercostal space.

Q25. Option B – Neoadjuvant chemotherapy.

T3 disease mandates neoadjuvant chemotherapy as per trials of FLOT and MAGIC regimes improving survival in patients with oesophageal cancer.

Q26. Option E – Plummer–Vinson syndrome.

Plummer–Vinson syndrome presents on the background of chronic anaemia and may show oesophageal webs and can also be associated with angular cheilitis. Pneumatic dilation is effective.

Q27. Option C – Intestinal type occurs in an older population than the diffuse type.

Intestinal-type gastric cancers have a higher male-to-female ratio, association with atrophic gastritis and are more likely well-differentiated with better prognosis. Diffuse gastric cancers are more likely poorly differentiated with signet cell findings and occur in a younger population with an equal male: female ratio.

Q28. Option C – Tyrosine kinase inhibitor.

Recurrence of GIST is managed by the tyrosine kinase inhibitor

Q29. Option C – T1a/T1b tumour.
    Endoscopic management can be considered for T1a tumours that are non-ulcerated, well-differentiated and 2 cm or less in size.

Q30. Option E – Sunitinib.
    Wild-type GISTs respond better to sunitinib.

Q31. Option B – Oesophageal cancer.
    A rat's tail appearance is seen in oesophageal cancer however this patient should have undergone a gastroscopy in the first instance. A bird's beak appearance is a typical barium swallow appearance in achalasia.

Q32. Option C – Switch to the paediatric scope and attempt six biopsies.
    Dilation risks perforation and narrow scope is the preferred course of action.

Q33. Option C – Urgent gastroscopy.
    Caustic injuries should have gastroscopy within 24 hours of ingestion to assess the injury and any later risks of perforation.

Q34. Option A – 24-hour pH Studies.
    Gastroscopy is performed to exclude malignancy and the presence of oesophagitis ± peptic stricture is sufficient to assume pathological reflux, whereas manometry studies are needed to assess motility as poor or absent motility can mean that anti-reflux surgery has poorly tolerated side effects of dysphagia.

Q35. Option E – Keep NBM and TPN.
    There are a number of ways this could be managed. OGD and feeding tube could be done but there would be a concern for disturbing the perforation. Conservative treatment with contrast swallow 7 days after the event is commonly successful. The patient should be kept NBM, with an NG tube on free drainage, IV PPI, antibiotics and antifungals. There is no consensus on oesophageal perforation management in terms of evidence-based but the MUSIOCS study may change this.

Q36. Option C – Book for emergency theatre for laparotomy and on-table gastroscopy.
    This patient has likely got stomach necrosis from incarcerated paraoesophageal hernia.

Q37. Option A – Gastroscopy.
    This patient should have undergone a gastroscopy for dysphagia, to begin with, the fixed narrowing gives concern for oesophageal cancer.

Q38. Option C – Protective ventilation and thoracic epidural analgesia.
    Thoracic epidural has been one of the most effective strategies to prevent post-op LRTI

Q39. Option D – Clip the vessel.
    Two modalities are advised in arresting bleeding endoscopically

Q40. Option C – His *H. pylori* status should be checked with a C13/14 breath test in 8 to confirm *H. pylori* eradication.

H. pylori status should be checked. Biopsies are not routinely taken during surgery for perforated duodenal ulcers. The C13/14 breath test can confirm eradication. Serum IgG levels cannot confirm eradication.

Q41. Option B – Downstage with imatinib.

This patient should receive the tyrosine kinase inhibitor imatinib in the hope of downstaging the disease in order to perform a limited gastric resection of the GIST.

Q42. Option B – POEM.

Overview POEM is effective for type 2 achalasia, laparoscopic cardiomyotomy is usually performed with a DOR fundoplication. Balloon dilatation has previously been shown to be as effective as laparoscopic cardiomyotomy but has reduced long-term efficacy.

Q43. Option B – Transhiatal oesophagectomy.

T1a disease would be suitable for EMR. Otherwise, resection is mandated. Node negative T1a can undergo transhiatal resection.

Q44. Option E – Ischaemic gastric conduit.

The right gastroepiploic artery

Q45. Option B – 10–12F tubes are optimal for feeding.

Fine bore tubes are preferred for feeding 5–8F. The position is ideally confirmed with pH testing. Acute variceal bleeding means. Long-term NG and NJ tubes should typically be changed every 4–6 weeks swapping them to the other nostril. Feeding jejunostomy or PEG tubes should be considered whenever a patient is likely to require feeding for more than 4–6 weeks.

Q46. Option E – Laparotomy and underrunning of ulcer.

Q47. Option E – Staging laparoscopy.

Staging laparoscopy can identify the peritoneal disease and metastatic spread not picked up by other staging modalities that would change the course of management.

Q48. Option D – Extrinsic compression.

Q49. Option E – Dysphagia lusoria.

Due to an aberrant right subclavian artery dysphagia, lusoria is a rare entity with the majority of patients being asymptomatic. Age-related reduced arterial compliance is thought to be the cause of symptoms.

Q50. Option B – Response to PPI.

Response to PPI has indicated a good response from anti-reflux surgery; however, those who do not respond to PPI therapy have been shown to respond well to surgery

Q51. Option D – Two pathologists have to confirm.

Q52. Option E – Carney syndrome.
Achalasia predisposes the patient to SCC up to 100× the expected population. Plummer–Vinson though rare is associated with SCC of the oesophagus, 3%–15% of the patients develop cancer of the oesophagus and pharynx. Obesity and reflux are related to oesophageal adenocarcinoma. The mechanism postulated involves transformation to Barrett's oesophagus. Carney triad comprises three tumours: gastric epithelioid leiomyosarcoma [later renamed gastrointestinal stromal tumour (GIST)], extra-adrenal paraganglioma, and pulmonary chondroma. Interestingly, in sporadic GIST, >1% have lymph node metastasis; in Carney, 25% have mets. Hence, in Carney, it is important to perform LN dissection. Though even with LN mets some are very indolent and some aggressive.

Q53. Option B – Alcohol.
FAP is not usually associated with gastric cancer; however, in the late stages, maybe, a key, endoscopic risk factor is associated with gastric cancer including carpeting of gastric polyps, solitary gastric polyps >20 mm and a polypoid mound of polyps. Gastric cancer patients also had a higher prevalence of gastric adenomas and fundic gland polyps with high-grade dysplasia.
Helicobacter is now declared a class 1 carcinogen for gastric cancer.
Reflux is more associated with junctional gastric cancers but by itself is not a risk factor.
Lynch syndrome is associated with gastric cancer 1%–13% of the time.
Meta-analysis showed that alcohol consumption elevated the risk of gastric cancer with an odds ratio (OR) of 1.39 (95% CI 1.20–1.61).

Q54. Option D – In type 3 tumours, one-third have died in 51 months.

Q55. Option D – Family history of ductal breast cancer and diffuse gastric cancer.
HDGC is a rare condition, usually identified with a mutation in the CGH1 gene. Patients to be screened include those whose person or family meets any of these criteria:
Families with two or more cases of stomach cancer, with at least one being diffuse gastric cancer
A person diagnosed with diffuse gastric cancer before the age of 40
Personal or family history of both diffuse gastric cancer and lobular breast cancer, if at least one person was diagnosed before age 50
Families with two or more cases of lobular breast cancer diagnosed before the age of 50
A person diagnosed with multiple different lobular breast cancers before the age of 50
A person with diffuse gastric cancer and a personal or family history of a cleft lip or cleft palate

Q56. Option D – PET scan.
PET scans are not useful in routine screening of gastric cancers as ⅓ are mucin-producing tumours and thus may have a false negative result. In selective cases, a PET scan would be useful

Q57. Option E – The treatment must be discussed in a multidisciplinary team.

Q58. Option A – Intraperitoneal chemotherapy.

Q59. Option E – Be discussed in a multidisciplinary team.

Q60. Option D – Has a higher reoperation rate.

Q61. Option A – Has a higher severe complication rate.

Q62. Option C – Removal of the primary tumour with two-phase lymphadenectomy.

Q63. Option B – Total gastrectomy.

Q64. Option D – Progressive dysphagia.
    The rest of the symptoms are common symptoms of non-oesophageal reflux symptoms. Progressive dysphagia is related to oesophageal cancer. In children with otitis media in children, 48.4% of them have pepsin/pepsinogen within the OM effusion. Though anti-reflux medication has not shown any benefit. Studies employing pH monitoring have shown a prevalence of GERD of 30%–65% among patients with asthma.

Q65. Option B – pH impedance manometry on PPI.
    The purpose of this test is to look for reflux, as the symptoms may be non-reflux related or sensitive oesophagus or even breakthrough reflux despite PPI. In pH impedance, the patient may be suffering non-acid reflux and thus symptoms are non-responsive to PPI

Q66. Option E – Under 3 hours.
    The half-life is less than 1 hour, and omeprazole is almost entirely cleared from plasma within 3–4 hours. Omeprazole is completely metabolised in the liver (Cederberg 1989)

Q67. Option D – Sucralfate.
    PPI, sucralfate, Gaviscon and bismuth require an acid environment to be activated

Q68. Option E – Raised intra-abdominal pressure.
    Raised intra-abdominal pressure increases the risk of reflux, the pressure differential between the thorax and abdomen is colloquially known as the thoracic pump, increasing reflux especially if the other continent measures are missing

Q69. Option E – Asymptomatically.
    The majority of hiatus hernias are asymptomatic. Though there is a high correlation between hiatus hernias and reflux, there are patients with the mechanism of reflux oesophagitis including other mechanisms of oesophageal continence and distal oesophageal clearance

Q70. Option D – Repair the crus with a mesh.

The role of the mesh remains unproven for standard use. There are no trials nor metanalyses or SR to support or refute use. This may be due to the diversity of meshes used, and hence, the data is clouded. There is some evidence to suggest the use of biologics.

Q71. Option C – Toupet has a better air swallowing side effect profile than Nissen.

Many meta-analysis show no difference in symptomatic reflux but improvement in gas complications.

Q72. Option D – Abnormal IRP and absent peristalsis.

This is the Chicago definition

Q73. Option A – Stapled cardioplasty.

In early achalasia, a radical procedure such as a stapled cardioplasty is not the primary procedure. The Botox injection into the GEJ may be used but is only indicated for frail patients whereby interventional therapy may be risky. The symptoms usually reoccur quickly after the Botox injection

Q74. Option D – Postoperative reflux.

Postoperative reflux in POEM is well recognised but felt to be clinically manageably in 20%–30% of patients

Q75. Option B – Endoscopy.

Any persistent dysphagia must be investigated for fear of missing cancer, i.e. secondary achalasia. However, after this, pH manometry is important to understand the barrier function remaining after myotomy, in cases of inadequate myotomy. Some patients have persistent symptoms due to absent peristalsis. The chest pain associated with type 3 achalasia can be persistent after surgery as this is due to the high oesophageal pressures not dealt with in the cardiomyotomy.

FURTHER READING

Cederberg C, Andersson T, Skånberg I. Omeprazole: pharmacokinetics and metabolism in man. *Scand J Gastroenterol Suppl.* 1989;166:33–40; discussion 41–42. doi: 10.3109/00365528909091241.

https://www.cancerresearchuk.org/about-cancer/neuroendocrine-tumours-nets/stomach-nets/types-grades

Ishigami H, Fujiwara Y, Fukushima R, Nashimoto A, Yabusaki H, Imano M, Imamoto H, Kodera Y, Uenosono Y, Amagai K, Kadowaki S, Miwa H, Yamaguchi H, Yamaguchi T, Miyaji T, Kitayama J. Phase III trial comparing intraperitoneal and intravenous paclitaxel plus S-1 versus cisplatin plus S-1 in patients with gastric cancer with peritoneal metastasis: PHOENIX-GC trial. *J Clin Oncol* 2018;36(19):1922–1929.

Lordick F, Mariette C, Haustermans K, Obermannová R, Arnold D; ESMO Guidelines Committee. Oesophageal cancer: ESMO Clinical Practice Guidelines for diagnosis, treatment and follow-up. *Ann Oncol* 2016;27(suppl 5):v50–v57. doi: 10.1093/annonc/mdw329.

Ludvigsson JF, Bai JC, Biagi F, et al. Diagnosis and management of adult coeliac disease: guidelines from the British Society of Gastroenterology. *Gut* 2014;63:1210–1228.

Miura MS, Mascaro M, Rosenfeld RM. Association between otitis media and gastroesophageal reflux: a systematic review. *Otolaryngol Head Neck Surg* 2012;146(3):345–352. doi: 10.1177/0194599811430809.

Morgagni P, Solaini L, Saragoni L, Monti M, Valgiusti M, Vittimberga G, Frassineti GL, Framarini M, Ercolani G. Conversion surgery in gastric cancer carcinomatosis. *Front Oncol* 2022;12:852559. doi: 10.3389/fonc.2022.852559.

Oor JE, Roks DJ, Koetje JH, Broeders JA, van Westreenen HL, Nieuwenhuijs VB, Hazebroek EJ. Randomized clinical trial comparing laparoscopic hiatal hernia repair using sutures versus sutures reinforced with non-absorbable mesh. *Surg Endosc* 2018;32(11):4579–4589. doi: 10.1007/s00464-018-6211-3.

Sgouros SN, Mpakos D, Rodias M, Vassiliades K, Karakoidas C, Andrikopoulos E, Stefanidis G, Mantides A. Prevalence and axial length of hiatus hernia in patients, with nonerosive reflux disease: a prospective study. *J Clin Gastroenterol* 2007;41(9):814–818. doi: 10.1097/01.mcg.0000225678.99346.65.

Siegal SR, Dolan JP, Hunter JG. Modern diagnosis and treatment of hiatal hernias. *Langenbecks Arch Surg* 2017;402(8):1145–1151. doi: 10.1007/s00423-017-1606-5.

Stephens MR, Lewis WG, Brewster AE, Lord I, Blackshaw GR, Hodzovic I, Thomas GV, Roberts SA, Crosby TD, Gent C, Allison MC, Shute K. Multidisciplinary team management is associated with improved outcomes after surgery for esophageal cancer. *Dis Esophagus* 2006;19(3):164–171. doi: 10.1111/j.1442-2050.2006.00559.x.

van Workum F, Verstegen MHP, Klarenbeek BR, Bouwense SAW, van Berge Henegouwen MI, Daams F, Gisbertz SS, Hannink G, Haveman JW, Heisterkamp J, Jansen W, Kouwenhoven EA, van Lanschot JJB, Nieuwenhuijzen GAP, van der Peet DL, Polat F, Ubels S, Wijnhoven BPL, Rovers MM, Rosman C; ICAN Collaborative Research Group. Intrathoracic vs cervical anastomosis after totally or hybrid minimally invasive esophagectomy for esophageal cancer: A randomized clinical trial. *JAMA Surg* 2021;156(7):601–610. doi: 10.1001/jamasurg.2021.1555.

8 Paediatric Surgery

Mike Kipling and Jigna Sheth

Q1. In the case of undescended testis, the primary objective of orchidopexy as early as possible is:
   A. Reduce the rate of testicular cancer
   B. Surgery is technically easier
   C. Reduced chance of testicular torsion
   D. Improved fertility later in life
   E. Reduced chance of anaesthetic complications

Q2. Lichen sclerosis of the foreskin
   A. Is most commonly diagnosed and treated by circumcision
   B. Is associated with hypospadias
   C. Is often treated with tacrolimus ointment
   D. Is often treated with prepuceplasty
   E. Is considered pre-malignant

Q3. Inguinal hernia repair in childhood usually employs:
   A. Lichtenstein technique
   B. Totally extraperitoneal (TEP) laparoscopic technique
   C. Bassini repair
   D. Ligation of the hernia sac (herniotomy)
   E. Shouldice technique

Q4. A 6-year-old child is on day 4 following a laparoscopic appendicectomy for mild, uncomplicated appendicitis with 3×5 mm ports (umbilical, hypogastric and left flank). The child fails to progress with diet and has diffuse abdominal pain. Blood parameters show a urea level of 35 mmol/L and a creatinine level of 350 µmol/L. You suspect the most likely cause to be:
   A. Renal failure from severe sepsis
   B. Ureteric ligation
   C. Upper GI bleeding
   D. Rhabdomyolysis
   E. Bladder injury

Q5. According to Advanced Paediatric Life Support guidelines, fluid boluses in children are usually:
   A. 10 mL/kg of warmed crystalloid in trauma
   B. 10 mL/kg of warmed crystalloid in sepsis
   C. 5 mL/kg of warmed crystalloid in trauma
   D. 10 mL/kg of packed red blood cells in trauma
   E. 20 mL/kg of warmed colloid in trauma

DOI: 10.1201/9781003221234-8

Q6. In paediatric trauma
   A.   Intraosseous access is contraindicated
   B.   Stiff cervical spine collars are recommended in addition to blocks and tape or manual in-line stabilisation
   C.   Children deteriorate early and steadily
   D.   Only recognised trauma units will ever have to deal with children with traumatic injuries
   E.   Splenic trauma is most often managed conservatively

Q7. Immediately life-threatening injuries in the early stages of paediatric trauma **do not** include:
   A.   Toxic shock syndrome
   B.   Tension pneumothorax
   C.   Cardiac tamponade
   D.   Open pneumothorax
   E.   Airway obstruction

Q8. Indications for considering the transfer of a child to a specialist burns unit **do not** include:
   A.   A partial thickness burn anywhere on the body with >2% body surface area (BSA) affected
   B.   A full-thickness burn of >1% BSA
   C.   Burns to special areas such as hands/face/neck/perineum/feet
   D.   Electrical burns
   E.   Consistent story and appropriate level of concern from parents

Q9. Epigastric hernias in children
   A.   Should be repaired laparoscopically
   B.   Rarely cause problems, so can often be managed conservatively
   C.   Usually contain the bowel
   D.   Are often associated with other congenital abnormalities
   E.   Are repaired using a mesh sublay technique

Q10. In children with symptomatic gallstones
   A.   The child should wait until they are old enough to see an adult upper GI surgeon before treatment
   B.   Open surgery is the standard of care
   C.   Conditions predisposing to gallstones include Crohn's disease and metabolic syndrome
   D.   Gallstones are most commonly seen in children with genetic syndromes
   E.   Gallstones are seen in around 1:1,000 children

Q11. Infantile pyloric stenosis most commonly presents
   A.   At 6–8 months of life
   B.   With vomiting and acidosis
   C.   With bilious vomiting
   D.   In female infants
   E.   At 6–8 weeks of life

Q12. In infantile pyloric stenosis
  A. The priority of management is surgery immediately after diagnosis to relieve the problem
  B. Correction of acid–base balance prior to surgery is less important than surgery as early as possible
  C. Is treated by endoscopic balloon dilatation of the pylorus
  D. Is treated by pyloroplasty involving seromuscular and mucosal layers
  E. Is treated by pyloromyotomy involving the seromuscular layer

Q13. Hirschprung's disease
  A. Is inherited via mostly recessive genes
  B. Is inherited via mostly dominant genes
  C. Is inherited by an X-linked recessive gene
  D. Mostly demonstrates a long aganglionic segment
  E. Mostly affects female children

Q14. A slim 2-year-old boy presents with an impalpable testicle on the right side, with the left side being normal. The next step in management should be:
  A. Ultrasound
  B. Beta-HCG treatment
  C. Clinical observation until puberty
  D. Laparoscopy ± Fowler–Stephen procedure, usually in a tertiary centre
  E. Referral to a clinical geneticist after surgery

Q15. Which of the below is not a cause of umbilical discharge in young people
  A. Urachal remnant
  B. Stitch sinus
  C. Branchial cyst
  D. Endometriosis
  E. Meckel's diverticulum

Q16. Anal fissure in children
  A. Is usually managed with 0.4% GTN ointment
  B. Is usually managed with anal Botox
  C. Is usually managed with diet, laxatives and reassurance
  D. Is usually secondary to sexual abuse
  E. Is usually secondary to underlying bowel pathology such as Crohn's disease

Q17. You are called by a general practitioner about a child with abdominal pain and diarrhoea, about whom the GP is concerned. The best course of action is:
  A. Diagnose gastroenteritis and advise pain relief/dioralyte in the community by phone
  B. Ask the GP to measure C-reactive protein and full blood count parameters and get back to you today
  C. Advise antibiotics and observation by the GP
  D. Ask the GP to arrange an urgent ultrasound scan
  E. Arrange to see and assess the child yourself

Q18. In blunt abdominal trauma in children
  A. CT is best avoided due to radiation risk even in the presence of a significant mechanism of injury
  B. Clinical signs are reliable markers of the severity of internal injuries
  C. A grade 4 splenic injury is always an indication for surgery
  D. A grossly unstable patient should always undergo surgery in a paediatric surgical unit
  E. Handlebar injuries can damage retroperitoneal structures such as the pancreas

Q19. In a child with ileocolic intussusception
  A. The management is with surgery
  B. The problem is mostly ileo-ileal
  C. The problem is mostly ileo-colonic
  D. The problem can wait until the morning for referral to a specialist following diagnosis in the evening
  E. The problem is caused by a pathological lead point in 80% of cases

Q20. An uncommon complication of circumcision is:
  A. Buried penis
  B. Iatrogenic epispadias
  C. Iatrogenic hypospadias
  D. Meatal stenosis
  E. Bleeding

Q21. In in-growing toenails in children
  A. Zadek's procedure is the first line
  B. Phenol is contraindicated
  C. Surgery is best performed under local anaesthesia
  D. Wedge excision±phenolisation is the most commonly employed technique
  E. The medial nail fold is most commonly affected

Q22. A 6-month-old infant presents with vomiting and intractable crying. Dance's sign is positive. The diagnosis is
  A. Testicular torsion
  B. Acute appendicitis
  C. Meckel's diverticulum perforation
  D. Intussusception
  E. Mid-gut volvulus

Q23. A 6-month-old boy presents with moderate right-sided scrotal swelling. Clinical examination confirms a hydrocoele. Your advice in the clinic is:
  A. Expectant management with observation and reassurance
  B. Ligation of patent processus vaginalis
  C. Jaboulay procedure
  D. Lord's procedure
  E. Aspiration under local anaesthetic

Q24. You are an adult surgeon with an interest in paediatric general surgery. A 9-year-old girl has been placed on your theatre list for excision of a cystic lump in the anterior triangle of her neck. It moves on the protrusion of the tongue. Your management is:
  A. Excision of the lump under a local anaesthetic
  B. Excision of the lump under a general anaesthetic
  C. Cancel surgery and referral to an ear, nose and throat specialist
  D. Urgent MRI of neck
  E. Incision and drainage of lump

Q25. Which of the following represents an item that is best extracted endoscopically from the stomach, rather than being allowed to pass once in that location:
  A. A coin
  B. A small toy car
  C. Safety razor head
  D. A button battery
  E. A single magnet

Q26. Formation of an ileoanal pouch in teenagers
  A. Should be deferred until adulthood by performing an ileostomy after colectomy for colitis or familial adenomatous polyposis.
  B. Should be performed by any colorectal surgeon.
  C. Should be performed by any specialist paediatric surgeon.
  D. Should involve discussion of future outcomes such as fertility and sexual function.
  E. Has the same rate of pouch failure when performed for ulcerative colitis as for Crohn's disease.

Q27. An infant presenting with an inguinal hernia at their baby check should have this repaired:
  A. As soon as possible
  B. At 6 months old
  C. At 12 months old
  D. Laparoscopically
  E. Using a Permacol mesh

ANSWERS

Q1. Option D – Improved fertility later in life.

British Association of Paediatric Surgery guidelines advocate surgery for undescended testis at an early age, around 12 months of life, for purposes of improved fertility later in life. The testicular cancer rate is only moderately reduced by orchidopexy but is thankfully vanishingly rare anyway. Surgery at an early age can be challenging due to the pubic fat pad, and anaesthetic risk diminishes with age. It may be that British guidance will change going forwards as worldwide guidelines are beginning to suggest surgery earlier, between 6 and 12 months of life for fertility purposes (European Society for Paediatric Urology and Canadian Association of Paediatric Surgeons). The British tendency to delay to 12 months is primarily driven by anaesthetic concerns.

Q2. Option A – Is most commonly diagnosed and treated by circumcision.

Lichen sclerosis of the foreskin is a benign, cryptogenic condition causing scarring of the foreskin and glans. Treatment is usually surgical, in all but mild cases, to prevent progression and damage to the glans and urinary meatus. However, steroid ointment and rarely tacrolimus ointment can be used in selected cases.

Q3. Option D – Ligation of the hernia sac (herniotomy).

Other than herniotomy, the above are all techniques employed in adult rather than paediatric patients. If laparoscopic techniques are employed to treat paediatric inguinal hernia, they usually involve trans-abdominal ligation of the hernia sac.

Q4. Option E – Bladder injury.

In children, the bladder sits higher out of the pelvis than it does in adults; hence, it is vulnerable both in trauma scenarios as well as with suprapubic ports in laparoscopic surgery. It is not uncommon for those more used to operating on adults to place the suprapubic port too low, inadvertently transgressing the bladder without knowledge of this at the time. Urea and creatinine rise due to peritoneal resorption. In simple appendicitis, anatomy should not be distorted enough to make ureteric ligation likely, and this should be vanishingly rare. Upper GI bleeding would create a urea rise but not a creatinine rise. Rhabdomyolysis would be an extremely rare complication of anaesthesia

Q5. Option A – 10 mL/kg of warmed crystalloid in trauma.

Generous fluid boluses of 20 mL/kg are employed in sepsis, but for the purposes of maintaining clot formation and avoiding haemodilution, this is reduced to 10 mL/kg in trauma and re-assessment of the situation. Boluses of blood are given at a volume of 5 mL/kg, all as per *APLS Manual Volume 6*.

Q6. Option E – Splenic trauma is most often managed conservatively.

While care should be taken to avoid growth plates, intraosseous access is often used in children with difficult intravenous access in a trauma situation. Hard cervical collars are no longer recommended, with manual in-line stabilisation or blocks and tape alone being as effective and not preventing other access to the head and neck or being as uncomfortable for the child, reducing compliance. Children will compensate for major injuries for a long time, before finally deteriorating precipitously, but liver and splenic injuries in children that would mandate surgery in adults can often be managed conservatively in a stable child with appropriate monitoring. Children are often brought by their parents/bystanders to the nearest hospital, rather than being brought by paramedics to a trauma centre, meaning that all general surgeons should be prepared to deal with such problems in extreme circumstances if it is not safe to transfer the child to a tertiary/trauma centre.

Q7. Option A – Toxic shock syndrome.

Toxic shock syndrome is a syndrome caused by a release of endotoxin and exotoxin occurring relatively late in trauma. The other pathologies can all cause an early threat to life in a traumatised child and are the key pathologies to identify early and manage to prevent rapid deterioration or demise of the child. Apart from toxic shock syndrome, these make up the key priorities in early trauma management in both advanced trauma life support and Advanced Paediatric Life Support algorithms.

Q8. Option E – Consistent story and appropriate level of concern from parents.

A–D are all indications to contact a burns unit for their consideration of transfer of the child for their assessment as per the Advanced Paediatric Life Support teaching. The latter scenario is not suggestive of non-accidental injury, suspicion of which should also prompt consideration of transfer.

Q9. Option B – Rarely causes problems, so can often be managed conservatively.

Mesh repairs are not usually employed in children, where a small incision and sutured repair are usually all that is required. These hernias rarely cause problems. Conservative management is a good option in the absence of symptoms or progressive enlargement of the hernia. They normally contain pre-peritoneal fat and emerge through tiny fascial defects.

Q10. Option C – Conditions predisposing to gallstones include Crohn's disease and metabolic syndrome.

Surgery should be laparoscopic wherever possible and should not be delayed until adulthood as this risks serious complications from gallstones such as pancreatitis. Gallstones in children in the United Kingdom are now seen most commonly in overweight but otherwise healthy children, with an incidence of around 1:100 according to Great Ormond Street Hospital figures. The surgery should be performed by a surgeon with sufficient expertise in cholecystectomy.

Q11. Option E – At 6–8 weeks of life.

Pyloric stenosis is more common in male infants, presenting around 6 weeks of life. It causes a metabolic hypochloraemic alkalosis via non-bilious vomiting.

Q12. Option E – Is treated by pyloromyotomy involving the seromuscular layer.

Infantile pyloric stenosis is most commonly seen in male infants around the age of 6 weeks of life. Acid–base defects should be corrected pre-operatively, as life-threatening apnoea can otherwise be seen. Surgery involves a pyloromyotomy, which can be performed using open or laparoscopic techniques. A complication to be avoided is entering the lumen of the pylorus, rather than leaving the mucosa intact as this runs the risk of leakage of gut contents and peritonitis – even when repaired.

Q13. Option B – Is inherited via mostly dominant genes.

Hirschprung's has an autosomal dominant inheritance pattern

Q14. Option D – Laparoscopy ± Fowler–Stephen procedure, usually in a tertiary centre.

If the testis is palpable in the groin, then the next step would be groin exploration; if the testis is not palpable, then it is not likely that the testis will be found in the groin at the time of exploration. An ultrasound does not change the fact that an operation is the appropriate next step. It should be performed by a surgeon who can perform both standard and Fowler–Stephen orchidopexy. In Europe, some infants are treated with beta-HCG to encourage testicular descent.

Q15. Option C – Endometriosis.

All of the above are causes of umbilical discharge seen in young people except branchial cysts, which cause neck lesions that can discharge if drained or ruptured due to infection.

Q16. Option C – Is usually managed with diet, laxatives and reassurance.

An anal fissure is not usually managed aggressively in children as it will almost always resolve with appropriate manipulation of stool and diet. Most are primary and simple, relating to constipation rather than serious secondary causes.

Q17. Option E – Arrange to see and assess the child yourself.

There is no substitute for a face-to-face clinical review of a child, particularly in the presence of concern from another professional. As children can present atypically, careful clinical assessment by an experienced clinician is important to ensure safe management.

Q18. Option E – Handlebar injuries can damage retroperitoneal structures such as the pancreas.

Due to their small size and flexibility versus adults, it is quite possible for handlebar injuries to create significant and deep injuries in children – this can include pancreatic transection, and this can be seen even in a reasonably well-looking child with minimal abdominal signs. CT should be used where appropriate in children if a significant injury is suspected. Many solid organ injuries that may demand operative management in an adult may be successfully managed conservatively in a child with appropriate monitoring. If a child is too unstable to safely transfer, a competent general surgeon should be used to stabilise the patient prior to transfer, such as laparotomy and abdominal packing to support resuscitation.

Q19. Option C – The problem is mostly ileo-colonic.

Ileocolic intussusception is most common and is usually managed by a hydrostatic reduction in the first instance with surgery being reserved for failure, perforation or peritonitis. It is a time-sensitive diagnosis and should be treated as such. If seen in children over 5 years, a pathological lead point becomes more likely, but before this, inflamed Peyer's patches are the most common cause.

Q20. Option B – Iatrogenic epispadias.

All of the above are relatively common complications of circumcision except for epispadias (an opening of the meatus onto the dorsum of the penis). While recognised, this is very rare and certainly not as common as iatrogenic hypospadias.

Q21. Option D – Wedge excision ± phenolisation is the most commonly employed technique.

Zadek's procedure, often with phenolisation, is the most aggressive surgical technique for managing in-growing toenails. Most children will undergo wedge excision of the lateral nail fold, with a local anaesthetic being reserved only for older children who felt compliant enough to safely complete the procedure in that manner.

Q22. Option D – Intussusception.

Dance's sign (empty right iliac fossa) is associated with a sausage-shaped mass in the abdomen are signs of ileo-colic intussusception.

Q23. Option A – Expectant management with observation and reassurance.

In most units, a hydrocoele would not be treated below the age of 2 years unless unusual circumstances exist. In an older child, ligation of patent processus would be an appropriate treatment, with 3–5 being treatments used only in adults.

Q24. Option C – Cancel surgery, referral to an ear, nose and throat specialist.

This scenario is concerning for a thyro-glossal cyst. The patient is likely to need a Sistrunk procedure, and as it is unlikely that you (as a general paediatric surgeon) will be competent to perform this in a child, an onward referral is usually appropriate. Pre-op workup will vary depending upon the treating clinician, so it is usually best to await their own management plan, rather than ordering investigations the patient may not need.

Q25. Option D – A button battery.

All of the above can potentially be safely allowed to pass through the GI tract of a child, except button batteries. Once past the cricopharyngeus in the neck, these will all usually pass on their own. If still in a position where they can be easily retrieved before passing into the small bowel, button batteries should be extracted endoscopically before a laparotomy becomes necessary. Magnets when multiple, or swallowed with other metallic objects, are again important to extract but are less of a problem when swallowed on their own.

Q26. Option D – Should involve discussion of future outcomes such as fertility and sexual function.

Formation of an ileostomy and exclusion of rectal function for any great period of time reduces the chance of good pouch function later in life. The counselling for this procedure is crucial and should encompass potential future functional issues. Pouch procedures are a specialist skill and should be performed by surgeons of either paediatric or colorectal specialism as long as they are regularly performing them in sufficient numbers to maintain their skills. Sometimes, this means collaborative working, which can also ease the transition to adult services later in life through familiarity. Pouch failure is significantly increased in Crohn's disease when compared to ulcerative colitis, and most surgeons consider this a contraindication to pouch surgery – though not all.

Q27. Option A – As soon as possible.

There is a little role in deferring inguinal herniotomy in neonates as complications such as incarceration are quite common and are sometimes difficult for parents to detect given the infant's limited means of communication. Prematurity may lead to delaying hernia surgery, particularly if associated with neonatal lung disease, but the British Association of Paediatric Surgeons' guidance is that the hernia should be repaired prior to discharge home if discovered following a baby check. Laparoscopic herniotomy is relatively uncommon, though is sometimes employed in specialist centres.

FURTHER READING

Bayreuther J, Wagener S, Woodford M, Edwards A, Lecky F, Bouamra O, Dykes E. Paediatric trauma: injury pattern and mortality in the UK. *Arch Dis Child Educ Pract Ed.* 2009 Apr;94(2):37–41. doi: 10.1136/adc.2007.132787.

Jobson M, Hall NJ. Current practice regarding the timing of patent processus vaginalis ligation for idiopathic hydrocele in young boys: a survey of UK surgeons. *Pediatr Surg Int.* 2017 Jun;33(6):677–681. doi: 10.1007/s00383-017-4085-4.

Mishra PK, Burnand K, Minocha A, Mathur AB, Kulkarni MS, Tsang T. Incarcerated inguinal hernia management in children: 'a comparison of the open and laparoscopic approach'. *Pediatr Surg Int.* 2014 Jun;30(6):621–624. doi: 10.1007/s00383-014-3507-9.

Tosounidis TH, Giannoudis PV. Paediatric trauma resuscitation: an update. *Eur J Trauma Emerg Surg.* 2016 Jun;42(3):297–301. doi: 10.1007/s00068-015-0614-9.

9 Peritoneal Malignancy

Alexios Tzivanakis and Brendan J. Moran

Q1. A 35-year-old man, who was previously fit and well, presented with acute appendicitis. He had an uneventful laparoscopic appendicectomy for non-perforated appendicitis. Histology was reported a few weeks later with a non-perforated low-grade appendiceal mucinous neoplasm (LAMN). What is the next step?
   A. Review the patient in OPD and offer laparoscopic right hemicolectomy
   B. Review the patient in OPD, organise colonoscopy and, if normal, discharge from the clinic
   C. Review the patient in OPD, organise colonoscopy and refer to a peritoneal malignancy centre for further advice
   D. Review the patient in OPD and refer to a peritoneal malignancy centre for further advice
   E. As it is a low-grade tumour, if there is no perforation, discharge from the clinic

Q2. A 50-year-old woman presented with acute appendicitis. She had a laparoscopic appendicectomy and at pathology had a 2.5 cm carcinoid (neuroendocrine tumour) in the specimen. What is the next step?
   A. Review the patient in OPD and offer laparoscopic right hemicolectomy.
   B. Review the patient in OPD and organise colonoscopy and, if normal, discharge from the clinic.
   C. Review the patient in OPD, and ask her what she wants?
   D. Review the patient in OPD and refer to a neuroendocrine (NET) centre for further advice prior to probably laparoscopic right hemicolectomy.
   E. Review patient in OPD and refer to a peritoneal malignancy centre for cytoreductive surgery and HIPEC.

Q3. A 53-year-old woman has been referred to the colorectal clinic under the 2-week wait pathway with a non-specific change of bowel habit. She is otherwise fit and well. Colonoscopy is incomplete due to significant discomfort. A CT colonoscopy is performed which shows no colonic pathology, but an abnormally dilated appendix containing fluid is identified. The rest of the peritoneal cavity and abdominal viscera are normal. She is referred to the colorectal MDT. What is the next step?
   A. Refer to the peritoneal malignancy unit for cytoreductive surgery and hyperthermic intraperitoneal chemotherapy.
   B. Diagnostic laparoscopy and, if there is no peritoneal disease, remove the appendix for histological diagnosis. If histology confirms an appendix tumour, proceed subsequently to a right hemicolectomy.
   C. Proceed to laparoscopic right hemicolectomy.
   D. Laparoscopy and, if there is no peritoneal disease, remove the appendix for histological diagnosis. Refer to the peritoneal malignancy unit for advice on further management.
   E. Percutaneous biopsy under interventional radiology.

DOI: 10.1201/9781003221234-9

Q4. A 43-year-old lady presented with acute appendicitis. Upon laparoscopy, there was a perforated appendix with some turbid fluid in RIF and pelvis. The appendix was gangrenous, and she has an uneventful appendicectomy and washout of the peritoneal cavity. Her histology came back, showing acute appendicitis with a perforation and a pT4 low-grade mucinous neoplasm of the appendix. How should she be managed from here on?

A. Offer colonoscopy and laparoscopic right hemicolectomy locally

B. Offer colonoscopy and do interval CT in 3–6 months to look for signs of pseudomyxoma peritonei

C. Offer colonoscopy and organise interval CT in 3–6 months and refer to the peritoneal malignancy unit for advice on surveillance

D. Offer colonoscopy and organise interval CT in 3–6 months and refer to the peritoneal malignancy unit for prophylactic cytoreductive surgery and HIPEC

E. Discharge from the clinic

Q5. A 47-year-old lady presents urgently to the gynaecological clinic with a suspected ovarian tumour. Three years previously, she had an appendicectomy for acute perforated appendicitis and the pathology showed an incidental low-grade appendix mucinous neoplasm (pT4). No further follow-up was performed after her appendicectomy. An USS of the pelvis and CT of the abdomen and pelvis showed a large $10 \times 15 \times 15$ cm right ovarian mass but otherwise normal. The gynaecology MDT asked for an opinion from the colorectal MDT for advice before proceeding with laparotomy, BSO and hysterectomy. Her CEA was 3, her CA 125 was 50 and her CA 199 was 210. What should the colorectal MDT advise?

A. Proceed with surgery as planned

B. Laparoscopy and, if no peritoneal disease is diagnosed, proceed with BSO and TAH

C. Colonoscopy and, if normal, proceed with BSO and TAH

D. Percutaneous biopsy

E. Colonoscopy and refer to a peritoneal malignancy unit for consideration for CRS and HIPEC as this likely represents a Krukenberg tumour from her prior appendix tumour

Q6. A 70-year-old man, otherwise fit and well, presents with acute appendicitis confirmed on a CT. The radiologist reported free fluid over the liver. At laparoscopy, he has an inflamed dilated, visually non-perforated, appendix with mucinous ascites in the right parabolic gutter, pelvis and over the liver. What should the surgeon do next?

A. Complete the appendicectomy, aspirate the ascites, send some for histology, wash the peritoneal cavity with warm water and refer to a peritoneal malignancy unit for CRS and HIPEC

B. Do a right hemicolectomy, aspirate the ascites, send some for histology, wash the peritoneal cavity with warm water and refer to a peritoneal malignancy unit for CRS and HIPEC

C. Do not remove the appendix, aspirate the ascites and send for histology, wash the peritoneal cavity with warm water and refer to a peritoneal malignancy unit for CRS and HIPEC

D. Do not remove the appendix, take biopsies and refer to a peritoneal malignancy unit for CRS and HIPEC

E. Abandon the procedure and refer to a peritoneal malignancy unit for CRS and HIPEC

Q7. A 46-year-old lady presented with anaemia and was diagnosed with caecal cancer. Her pre-operative staging was clear. She had an uneventful laparoscopic right hemicolectomy. Her histology confirmed a pT4N1M0 moderately differentiated mucinous adenocarcinoma of the caecum. She had adjuvant chemotherapy. On her first surveillance scan 1-year post-op, she was found to have a large right adnexal cystic mass 10×1×6 cm. The CT was otherwise normal. Her CEA, CA-125 and CA-199 were normal. What is the recommended next step?

A. Refer her to the regional gynae-oncology MDT as this is probably an ovarian cancer

B. Refer her to a gynaecologist for excision of this mass

C. Refer her for systemic chemotherapy and then discuss with a peritoneal malignancy centre for CRS and HIPEC

D. Refer to a peritoneal malignancy centre for consideration of CRS and HIPEC as this is most likely a Krukenberg tumour from her pT4 cancer

E. Excise the ovary

Q8. A 60-year-old man, previously fit and well, presents with anaemia. A colonoscopy confirms a large annular caecal tumour. He is subsequently admitted whilst awaiting a staging CT. Admission CT confirms a large caecal mass, small bowel obstruction, and several omental deposits and non-specific nodularity along the right paracolic gutter. An isolated liver metastasis was noted. The chest CT was normal. What should be the next step?

A. Laparotomy, right hemicolectomy and omentectomy followed by adjuvant chemotherapy

B. Laparoscopy, accurate assessment of peritoneal disease, loop ileostomy, liver MRI, referral to oncology and discussion with a peritoneal malignancy centre for combined CRS and HIPEC with liver metastasectomy after chemotherapy and restaging

C. Laparoscopy, accurate assessment of peritoneal disease burden, loop ileostomy, liver MRI and referral to peritoneal malignancy centre for combined CRS and HIPEC with liver metastasectomy

D. Laparotomy, right hemicolectomy and referral to peritoneal malignancy centre for consideration of CRS and HIPEC followed by chemotherapy and liver resection

E. Laparotomy, right hemicolectomy, liver MRI and systemic chemotherapy followed by liver resection

Q9. A 60-year-old lady, who is otherwise fit and well, had a laparoscopic left hemicolectomy for a pT4N0M0 colon tumour. She did not have any adjuvant chemotherapy after her surgery and is now under surveillance. Her first-year CT was clear but her CEA has risen to above normal at 18 months. CT of the chest and liver were normal. There were several omental nodules and two 10 and 12-mm nodules in the left iliac fossa. What should be the recommendation of the colorectal MDT?

A. Laparoscopy/-tomy locally and excise the affected areas
B. Refer to oncology for palliative chemotherapy
C. Refer to oncology for systemic chemotherapy
D. Refer to the peritoneal malignancy centre for advice and consideration of CRS and HIPEC
E. Continue surveillance

Q10. A 70-year-old fit and independent man was diagnosed with colonic cancer 2 years ago and had a laparoscopic right hemicolectomy for a T4N1M0 poorly differentiated colonic tumour. He had adjuvant chemotherapy and had his first annual surveillance CT at 1 year which reported no detectable disease. A subsequent CT a year later reported two peritoneal nodules in the right iliac fossa. He was restarted on chemotherapy. His mid-chemotherapy CT showed a reduction in the two known nodules and a new omental nodule. He was changed to a different chemotherapy regimen and a subsequent CT at 6 months confirmed a sustained response with no new disease sites seen. What should be the recommendation of the MDT?

A. Laparoscopy locally, and if no other disease is found, excise the areas of disease
B. Continue with maintenance systemic chemotherapy and restage in 6 months
C. Continue systemic chemotherapy and refer to peritoneal malignancy centre for consideration of CRS and HIPEC after laparoscopy
D. Refer for a cyber knife of these lesions
E. Stop chemotherapy and restage

ANSWERS

Q1. Option C – Review patient in OPD, organise colonoscopy and refer to a peritoneal malignancy centre for further advice.

An incidental finding of a LAMN in an appendix specimen following resection for a non-perforated appendicitis is uncommon. This patient has a low risk of developing pseudomyxoma peritonei (progressive mucinous ascites). Risks are higher if there is mucin or abnormal cells outside the appendix. These tumours rarely metastasise to the lymph nodes, and therefore, prophylactic right hemicolectomy is not advised or indicated. However, there is a chance of synchronous colonic pathology (1%–4%), and therefore, a colonoscopy should generally be performed once the patient has recovered from surgery. The patient should be referred to a peritoneal malignancy unit for a review of pathology slides and recommendations for follow-up. Generally, follow-up is by regular radiological imaging (CT or MRI of the abdomen/pelvis at years 1, 3, 5 and 10 years) and tumour marker measurement (CEA, CA-125 and CA-199) at the time of imaging.

Q2. Option D – Review the patient in OPD and refer to a neuroendocrine (NET) centre for further advice prior to probably laparoscopic right hemicolectomy.

Approximately 1% of all appendix specimens have an associated tumour, the majority being carcinoids (neuroendocrine tumours) with the second most common being epithelial tumours. Tumours up to 1 cm in size generally require no further intervention; tumours greater than 2 cm, involving the meso-appendix or resection margin or other high-risk pathological features should be considered for right hemicolectomy after advice from a NET MDT to assess the nodal status

Q3. Option D – Laparoscopy and if no peritoneal disease, remove the appendix for histological diagnosis. Refer to the peritoneal malignancy unit for advice on further management.

The majority of these tumours will be a LAMN. In the majority of cases, the recommended treatment is appendicectomy. The patient has a low risk of developing pseudomyxoma peritonei (PMP) (progressive gross mucinous ascites). PMP tumours rarely metastasise to the lymph nodes or systemically, and therefore, prophylactic right hemicolectomy is not advised or indicated. If the histology shows a high-grade mucinous neoplasm of the appendix, an adenocarcinoma or a goblet cell appendix adenocarcinoma of the appendix, then the patient should be referred to a peritoneal malignancy unit for advice and for consideration of cytoreductive surgery (CRS) and HIPEC which will involve a right parietal peritonectomy, right hemicolectomy, greater omentectomy and HIPEC, and bilateral oophorectomy. The chance of finding peritoneal disease and involved lymph nodes at CRS and HIPEC is about 20% and just under 20%, respectively.

Q4. Option C – Offer colonoscopy and organise interval CT in 3–6 months and refer to the peritoneal malignancy unit for advice on surveillance.

An incidental finding of a LAMN in an appendix specimen following resection is uncommon. The patient is at low risk of developing PMP, though risks are higher if there are cells or mucin outside the appendix. These tumours rarely metastasise to the lymph nodes, and therefore, prophylactic right hemicolectomy is not advised or indicated. However, there is a small risk of significant synchronous colonic pathology (1%–4%), and therefore, a colonoscopy is recommended once the patient has recovered from surgery. In view of the perforation, an interval CT may help to assess the peritoneal cavity for abnormalities and act as a baseline. The patient should be referred to a peritoneal malignancy unit for pathology review by an expert pathologist. If the interval CT is clear, she should be followed up by regular radiological imaging (CT or MRI of the abdomen/pelvis at 1, 3, 5 and 10 years) and sequential measurement of tumour markers (CEA, CA-125 and CA-199).

Q5. Option E – Colonoscopy and refer to a peritoneal malignancy unit for consideration for CRS and HIPEC as this likely represents a Krukenberg tumour from her prior appendix tumour.

This lady most likely has a Krukenberg tumour secondary to a previous T4 low-grade mucinous appendix tumour. She should be referred to a peritoneal malignancy centre, a colonoscopy should be performed. Optimal treatment may require CRS and HIPEC. It is likely that there is a further mucinous disease not visualised in imaging. Pelvic peritonectomy is more difficult, complex and dangerous if the planes have been disturbed by a prior BSO and TAH.

Q6. Option A – Complete appendicectomy, aspirate the ascites and send it for histology, wash the peritoneal cavity with warm water and refer to a peritoneal malignancy unit for CRS and HIPEC.

This patient has PMP, most likely from a perforated appendix neoplasm. Removing the appendix will provide histology (most likely low-grade) and will treat his acute appendicitis. He should have a colonoscopy once he has recovered from his operation to exclude a colonic tumour or a significant polyp and then be referred to a peritoneal malignancy unit. There are two options available to the patient. One is to proceed with CRS and HIPEC or adopt a watch-and-wait policy. This is dependent on patient preference and volume of disease on an interval CT at 3–6 months post-op.

Q7. Option D – Refer to a peritoneal malignancy centre for consideration of CRS and HIPEC as this is most likely a Krukenberg tumour from her pT4 cancer.

This lady had a pT4 tumour which increases the risk of developing peritoneal metastasis. She most likely has a Krukenberg tumour, secondary to her prior colon cancer. Urgent referral to a peritoneal malignancy centre is recommended for consideration for CRS and HIPEC involving, at a minimum, pelvic peritonectomy, bilateral salpingo-oophorectomy and greater omentectomy followed by HIPEC. The risk of synchronous or metachronous contra-lateral ovarian involvement is in the region of 80%. Systemic chemotherapy may not control Krukenberg tumours as the ovary, like the brain, in many patients appears to be a "sanctuary" site from the effects of systemically administered chemotherapy.

Rapid ovarian enlargement may occur and urgent surgery may be needed.

Q8. Option B – Laparoscopy, accurate assessment of peritoneal disease, loop ileostomy, liver MRI and referral to oncology and discussion with peritoneal malignancy centre for combined CRS and HIPEC with liver metastasectomy after chemotherapy and restaging.

Laparoscopy, if feasible, will allow assessment of the peritoneal disease using the peritoneal carcinomatosis index (PCI). PCI is a composite of lesion size (1–3 based on the size of the deposits) and 13 abdominal anatomical sites. These 13 sites comprise 9 for the peritoneal cavity itself, right upper and lower, right flank, pelvis, left upper and lower, left flank, central and epigastrium and 4 for the small bowel (upper and lower jejunum and ileum). The PCI ranges from 0 to 39. As expected, the lower the PCI, the more likely that a complete tumour removal is achievable and the better the prognosis. Very high PCIs (>20) may not benefit from CRS and HIPEC, and morbidity may exceed the benefit. Loop ileostomy will resolve the obstruction. This patient has contained peritoneal disease but also has the systemic disease. The optimal treatment is systemic chemotherapy, if tolerated, with subsequent imaging. Limited liver resection can be performed in conjunction with CRS and HIPEC in selected cases.

Q9. Option D – Refer to the peritoneal malignancy centre for advice and consideration of CRS and HIPEC.

This lady had a pT4 tumour which increases her risk of developing a peritoneal disease. She has not had any systemic chemotherapy and has developed the peritoneal disease over 18 months. Optimal prognosis is seen in patients with a long interval time between primary and metastatic disease. Additionally, as for many diseases, a period of stability, or response, to systemic chemotherapy prior to CRS and HIPEC is generally associated with a better prognosis. A diagnostic staging laparoscopy prior to her CRS and HIPEC is recommended to confirm the distribution of the disease. The peritoneal malignancy unit may recommend an upfront diagnostic laparoscopy prior to, and after, systemic chemotherapy. A laparoscopy will help to assess the peritoneal disease distribution using the PCI as outlined above.

Q10. Option C – Continue systemic chemotherapy and refer to the peritoneal malignancy centre for consideration of CRS and HIPEC after laparoscopy.

This gentleman had a T4N1 tumour and therefore is at risk of both peritoneal and systemic recurrence. He has had a peritoneal disease that progressed while on systemic chemotherapy. However, he responded to second-line systemic treatment. His imaging suggests localised and limited disease, but biologically, his disease is aggressive, as evident from the poor differentiation and the fact that it progressed while having systemic chemotherapy. However, stabilisation on second-line chemotherapy and a trial of time for other metastatic diseases suggest that he might benefit from CRS and HIPEC. Surgeons at a peritoneal malignancy centre would consider diagnostic laparoscopy prior to listing for CRS and HIPEC to confirm the distribution of disease and to try and rule out low-volume diffuse disease not seen on imaging.

FURTHER READING

Bijelic L, Ramos I, Goeré D. The Landmark Series: surgical treatment of colorectal cancer peritoneal metastases. *Annals of Surgical Oncology*. 2021 May 9:1–1.

Govaerts K, Lurvink RJ, De Hingh IH, Van der Speeten K, Villeneuve L, Kusamura S, Kepenekian V, Deraco M, Glehen O, Moran BJ, Barrios-Sanchez P. Appendiceal tumours and Pseudomyxoma peritonei: literature review with PSOGI/EURACAN clinical practice guidelines for diagnosis and treatment. *European Journal of Surgical Oncology*. 2021 Jan 1;47(1): 11–35.

Mehta A, Mittal R, Chandrakumaran K, Carr N, Dayal S, Mohamed F, Moran B, Cecil T. Peritoneal involvement is more common than nodal involvement in patients with high-grade appendix tumors who are undergoing prophylactic cytoreductive surgery and hyperthermic intraperitoneal chemotherapy. *Diseases of the Colon & Rectum*. 2017 Nov 1;60(11):1155–1161.

Mehta AM, Bignell MB, Alves S, Dayal SP, Mohamed F, Cecil TD, Moran BJ. Risk of ovarian involvement in advanced colorectal or appendiceal tumors involving the peritoneum. *Diseases of the Colon & Rectum*. 2017 Jul 1;60(7):691–696.

Murphy EM, Farquharson SM, Moran BJ. Management of an unexpected appendiceal neoplasm. *Journal of British Surgery*. 2006 Jul;93(7):783–792.

10 Robotic Surgery

James Royle, Peter Vaughan-Shaw,
Nicholas T. Ventham, Golam Farook,
and Stephen Holtham

Q1. Regarding robotic-assisted surgical procedures, which one of the following statements is untrue?
   A. The camera arm is directly controlled by the surgeon
   B. Endowrist instruments generally afford 7 degrees of freedom
   C. The ROLARR trial demonstrated significantly reduced conversion rates with robotic-assisted anterior resection compared to laparoscopic cases
   D. Robotic-assisted surgery has a shorter learning curve than laparoscopic surgery
   E. Robotic-assisted surgery is considered safe when performed by an experienced surgeon

Q2. A 78-year-old woman with a history of ischaemic heart disease and COPD is undergoing a robotic-assisted anterior resection. After stapling across the IMA, there is evidence of a brisk bleed from the root of the vessel and the camera view is rapidly obscured by blood. After informing your ST2 assistant and the wider theatre team of this, what would be the best immediate management for this patient?
   A. Continue robot-assisted surgery
   B. Convert to traditional laparoscopy
   C. Ask the theatre staff to contact the industry representative about a potential stapler mis-fire
   D. Perform standard undocking and convert to open surgery
   E. Perform emergency undocking and convert to open surgery

Q3. Regarding robotic-assisted surgical procedures, which one of the following statements is true?
   A. Port positioning for robotic-assisted anterior resection is the same as for laparoscopic anterior resection
   B. Artificial intelligence (AI) is generally used
   C. Telesurgery is generally used, allowing the surgeon to be in a different city or hospital
   D. A recoverable fault does not generally require a restart of the robotic system
   E. Improved tactile feedback enhances surgical precision

DOI: 10.1201/9781003221234-10

Q4. A 68-year-old man undergoes a robotic-assisted abdominal wall hernia repair and goes home the same day. Forty-eight hours later, he presents to A&E generally well with pyrexia. His white cell count is 18.5×10^9/L, and he has nonspecific abdominal pain and tenderness. What is the next appropriate step in his management?
A. Conservative treatment with IV fluids and observation
B. Diagnostic laparotomy
C. Diagnostic laparoscopy
D. CT abdomen/pelvis with IV contrast
E. Robotic-assisted exploration of the abdomen

Q5. Which of the following is not considered a key component in CME surgery?
A. Dissection in the correct embryological plane
B. Central venous ligation
C. D2 lymphadenectomy
D. D3 lymphadenectomy
E. D4 lymphadenectomy

Q6. Which of the following is not considered one of the four main pelvic lymph node stations relevant to rectal cancer?
A. Common iliac
B. External iliac (proximal + distal)
C. Internal iliac (proximal + distal)
D. Obturator
E. Inguinal

Q7. Which of the following is not considered an advantage of the present widely available robotic systems?
A. Stable viewing platform
B. Three-dimensional vision
C. Multiple arm retraction
D. Haptic feedback
E. Wristed instrumentation

Q8. A 50-year-old lady with no comorbidities and a BMI of 35 undergoes a difficult robot-assisted low anterior resection for rectal cancer. The procedure takes 8 hours. In recovery she complains of some left leg pain and by the following morning has a tense calf and paraesthesia foot. No pulses are palpable in the foot. What is the likely diagnosis?
A. Deep venous thrombosis
B. Compartment syndrome
C. Chronic arterial ischaemia
D. Neuropraxia
E. Meralgia paresthetica

Q9. A case of a robotic right hemicolectomy with complete mesocolic excision (CME) of central D3 lymph node stations is being performed. During the procedure, there is sudden and catastrophic bleeding. Which of the following statements is not true:

A. The relationship between the superior mesenteric vein and ileocolic artery is highly consistent

B. Bleeding can occur catastrophically from the Henle trunk, with branches of the right gastroepiploic vein, superior right colic vein, anterior superior pancreaticoduodenal vein and right colic artery having variable anatomy and insertion

C. Relevant lymph node stations in right hemicolectomy include 223, 213 and 203

D. Profuse uncontrolled bleeding may require kocherisation of the duodenum or the Cattell–Brasasch manoeuvre to control the proximal SMV

E. Blind suture ligation may exacerbate the bleeding and risks damage to the SMV and compromise to the small bowel vascularity

ANSWERS

Q1. Option C – The ROLARR trial demonstrated significantly reduced conversion rates with robotic-assisted anterior resection compared to laparoscopic cases

This statement is **untrue**. The ROLARR trial demonstrated significantly reduced conversion rates with robotic-assisted anterior resection compared to laparoscopic cases

In established robotic systems, the camera arm is generally controlled by the surgeon via the surgeon console. During docking, the camera will be manually controlled like in conventional laparoscopy. However, once docked, the operating surgeon controls the camera, which ensures that they can direct and zoom as needed.

Established robotic instruments may allow as many as 7 degrees of freedom – rotation, in/out, pitch, yaw, wristed yaw, grasp, and wristed pitch. In open surgery, you can achieve what might be described as 6 (free motion) degrees of freedom (DoFs), and this is reduced to 4 degrees with conventional (i.e. non-articulating) laparoscopic instruments. DoFs are often described using nautical terminologies such as pitch (tilting in a vertical vector), yaw (turning to the left or right) and roll (tilting from side to side).

The ROLARR trial was a multicentre RCT of robotic-assisted vs. laparoscopic surgery for rectal cancer resection where the primary end point was conversion to open laparotomy. Four hundred seventy-one patients were recruited. The overall rate of conversion to open laparotomy was 10.1%: 19 of 236 patients (8.1%) in the robotic-assisted laparoscopic group and 28 of 230 patients (12.2%) in the conventional laparoscopic group (unadjusted risk difference=4.1% [95% CI, −1.4% to 9.6%]; adjusted odds ratio=0.61 [95% CI, 0.31–1.21]; $P=0.16$)

The conversion rate was lower than expected in the conventional lap group, perhaps due to the increasing experience of the surgeons taking part. However, differences were apparent in the conversion rates for the conventional and robotic-assisted laparoscopic groups in men, with robotic-assisted laparoscopic surgery appearing to offer a benefit – perhaps due to the narrower male pelvis with more operator-controlled retraction, better optics, and instrument precision in robotic cases.

Learning curves have been shown to be shorter for robotic-assisted procedures. There is no fulcrum effect and movements more closely replicate the surgeon, and those movements are performed in open surgery.

Q2. Option E – Perform emergency undocking and convert to open surgery

There are some clues to the safest answer in the stem. First, the patient has a number of comorbidities which means the risk that bleeding might rapidly impact her physiology is increased. Second, the view is immediately obscured so you cannot continue and need to either clean the camera or convert. Third, you have a relatively junior assistant who may not be able to rapidly exchange and clean the camera and simultaneously operate the sucker. Robotic systems can be rapidly undocked in emergencies and such procedures must be learnt by both surgeons and theatre staff.

Q3. Option D – A recoverable fault does not generally require a restart of the robotic system

Port positioning differs from robotic surgery due to the absence of the fulcrum effect and the increased ability to work in smaller spaces (and with ports closer together). Port positions will vary between robotic platforms.

AI is not yet established as an adjunct to robotic-assisted surgery. It is possible that in the future AI may provide the surgeon with clues to anatomy and pathology, and early warning messages e.g., if instruments are in danger of damaging a structure.

Telesurgery describes the remote operation of the robotic system. Telesurgery is a real concept with the emergence of robotic surgery. However, it is not the norm, and the operating surgeon is predominantly present in the operating room. Of course, this provides important safety in case of robotic malfunction or the need to convert. Nevertheless, telesurgery has been performed and provides the following potential benefits:

1. Provides high-quality surgery to medically underserved locations such as rural areas, battlefields, and spacecraft.
2. Eliminates the need for long-distance travel, along with travel-related financial burden and dangers.
3. 3-Dimensional display system provides shared, high-definition visual feedback to surgeons at different centres simultaneously.
4. Allows for surgical collaboration amongst surgeons at different medical centres in real time.

Q4. Option D – CT abdomen/pelvis with IV contrast

Just as with a laparoscopic procedure, there is a risk of iatrogenic bowel injury with robotic-assisted surgery. In theory, this may be increased compared to conventional laparoscopy due to the absence of tactile feedback from the instruments, and as such, it is imperative that instruments are kept within the surgeon's view at all times. In this question, the patient would not expect to be this unwell following a simple day-case hernia repair. As such, he has a bowel injury until proven otherwise. If he was unstable, then diagnostic laparoscopy may be the most appropriate option, but with rapid CT now available at the front door of most surgical units, this may provide reassurance that there is not a major post-operative complication. Of course, even if the scan appears normal, this does not completely rule out a complication requiring a return to the theatre. If a return to the theatre was required, whether a diagnostic laparoscopy or laparotomy was most appropriate would depend on the skill set and set-up of the surgical unit in question and the evolving condition of the patient.

The development of robotic techniques in colorectal cancer has opened new possibilities in terms of more radical but minimally invasive surgery.

Q5. Option D – D3 lymphadenectomy

CME should be considered in three components: (1) Dissection in the correct embryological plane (e.g., Toldt's fascia) (2) Central venous ligation (taking the ileocolic at or near its origin) (3) D2 (e.g. ileocolic) vs. D3 (e.g. SMV) lymphadenectomy. Most colorectal cancer surgeons will always apply elements 1 and 2, D3 lymphadenectomy is usually reserved for selected patients with suspected pathological lymph nodes identified on preoperative imaging. CT 3D reconstructions can be used to guide surgeons. Potential benefits are a lower risk of local recurrence and greater long-term disease-specific survival. Risks are greater for significant haemorrhage that can be catastrophic (especially venous bleeding around or from the veins of Henle or the SMV). Current literature does not convincingly justify applying this to all patients.

Q6. Option E – Inguinal

Inguinal nodes are typically seen in anal cancer.

CT PET can be used to confirm involved nodes identified on pelvic MRI. Literature indicates that MRI tends to over-stage lymph nodes, so PET is a useful adjunct and interval re-staging post-chemo-radiotherapy can also indicate if nodes were involved if they responded to DXT.

Pelvic LND is an advanced technique practised laparoscopically for some years in Japan; improved local recurrence reported in the literature did not transform towards universal practice. However, robotic platforms might change that; it would be prudent to seek out a urological robotic surgeon colleague with that skill set and experience who might be able to partner in such cases.

The development of robotic techniques in colorectal cancer has opened new possibilities in terms of more radical but minimally invasive surgery.

Q7. Option D – Haptic feedback

Whilst several of the leading robotic platforms are aiming to develop this technology, haptic feedback is not currently a feature of most of the presently available systems. Haptic feedback, the conveyance of forces, motion or vibration patterns to the user, is an important aspect of all surgery including open and to a lesser extent laparoscopic surgery. As such, most robotic surgery relies on visual feedback, for example, the use of visual cues to determine whether tissue is under tension. Robotic console operators must be particularly careful of the force applied to the tissue and particularly off-camera instruments.

Q8. Option B – Compartment syndrome

This lady has undergone a prolonged procedure whilst in the lithotomy (or Lloyd–Davies) steep head-down position. She has developed compartment syndrome; increased intracompartmental pressure within a closed osteofascial compartment, causing impairment of local circulation. Her obesity is an additional risk factor. Without prompt identification and decompression (fasciotomy), she would be at risk of amputation. As with all surgery, careful patient positioning with due attention to at-risk bony prominences is critically important. During long robotic procedures, a scheduled leg rest is usually performed.

Common peroneal nerve neuropraxia is a relatively common (15.8%) occurrence, and like DVT, it would not explain the lack of pulses on examination. Given her lack of vascular risk factors and the acuity of the presentation, chronic arterial ischaemia is less likely. Likewise, meralgia paresthetica, compression of the lateral cutaneous nerve of the thigh, would cause numbness on the outer aspect of the thigh.

Q9. Option A – The relationship between the superior mesenteric vein and ileocolic artery is highly consistent

The relationship between the SMV and ileocolic artery is highly variable. The SMV is mostly anterior to the ileocolic artery (57%) but can be posterior (43%). Furthermore, the right colic artery, where present, is more commonly anterior to the SMV (90%) and less frequently posterior (10%). Intimate anatomical knowledge is critically important when performing more radical procedures such as CME right hemicolectomy. The bleeding complications of such procedures are higher (Bertelsen BJS 2016). The Henle trunk is a site of potential haemorrhage close to the pancreas and duodenum with branches listed. Suitable operative procedures may be required in the extremis, and enlisting the expert assistance of a colleague, especially from vascular, HPB or transplant subspecialties may be lifesaving. Blind suturing risks injuring or ligating the SMV and the resulting venous ischaemia can cause loss of the entire small bowel.

FURTHER READING

Bertelsen CA, Neuenschwander AU, Jansen JE, Kirkegaard-Klitbo A, Tenma JR, Wilhelmsen M, Rasmussen LA, Jepsen LV, Kristensen B, Gögenur I; Copenhagen Complete Mesocolic Excision Study (COMES); Danish Colorectal Cancer Group (DCCG). Short-term outcomes after complete mesocolic excision compared with 'conventional' colonic cancer surgery. *Br J Surg*. 2016 Apr;103(5):581–589. doi: 10.1002/bjs.10083. Epub 2016 Jan 18. PMID: 26780563.

Choi PJ, Oskouian RJ, Tubbs RS. Telesurgery: Past, present, and future. *Cureus*. 2018;10(5):e2716. doi:10.7759/cureus.2716

Hillel AT, Kapoor A, Simaan N, Taylor RH, Flint P. Applications of robotics for laryngeal surgery. *Otolaryngol Clin North Am*. 2008 Aug;41(4):781–791, vii. doi: 10.1016/j.otc.2008.01.021

Jayne D, Pigazzi A, Marshall H, et al. Effect of robotic-assisted vs conventional laparoscopic surgery on risk of conversion to open laparotomy among patients undergoing resection for rectal cancer: The ROLARR Randomized Clinical Trial. *JAMA*. 2017;318(16):1569–1580.

Kumar P, Ravi B. 2019. A comparative study of robots in laparoscopic surgeries. In *Proceedings of the Advances in Robotics* 2019 (AIR 2019). Association for Computing Machinery, New York, NY, Article 14, 1–6.

Leijte E, de Blaauw I, Van Workum F, et al. Robot assisted versus laparoscopic suturing learning curve in a simulated setting. *Surg Endosc*. 2020;34:3679–3689.

Livinti I, et al. Laparoscopic versus robotic surgery learning curves. *J Minim Invasive Gynecol*. 2015;22(6):S8–S9.

Okamura AM. Haptic feedback in robot-assisted minimally invasive surgery. *Curr Opin Urol*. 2009;19:102–107.

Pridgeon S, Bishop CV, Adshead J. Lower Limb Compartment Syndrome as a complication of robot-assisted radical prostatectomy: the UK experience. *BJUI*. 2013;112(4):485–488.

Sanchez-Margallo FM, Sanchez-Margallo JA. Ergonomics in laparoscopic surgery. In: Malik AM (Ed.), *Laparoscopic Surgery*. London: IntechOpen; Feb 2017. https://www.intechopen.com/chapters/52944 doi: 10.5772/66170

11 Statistics

Muhammad Rafay Sameem Siddiqui
and Sarah Abdelbar

Q1. A diagnostic study investigating colonoscopy versus CT to identify sigmoid tumours is conducted. A total of 500 patients are recruited and 10 cancers are identified and biopsied. The CT identifies seven of these tumours and one area of thickening in the caecum. What would the sensitivity of the index investigation be?
- A. 70%
- B. 88%
- C. 99%
- D. 80%
- E. 48%

Q2. A 54-year-old patient is admitted with gallstone pancreatitis. An MRCP shows no stones in the CBD but a dilated CBD. An intraoperative ultrasound suggests a CBD, stone but an intraoperative cholangiogram is clear. If the sensitivity and positive predictive value of intraoperative USS are 85% and 70%, respectively, what number of patients would have an unnecessary cholangiogram in a sample of 50 patients of whom 60% had CBD stones on MRI?
- A. 20
- B. 11
- C. 17
- D. 5
- E. 8

Q3. A meta-analysis is conducted on the management of cholecystitis with or without antibiotics. Seven studies are included comparing broad-spectrum antibiotics versus no antibiotics. The demographic data included age, sex, race and duration of symptoms. The p-value was significant in three of four of these parameters. A fixed-effect model looking at significant morbidity was 2.6 [1.8–3.9] in favour of antibiotics. What is the least accurate statement about these results?
- A. There is likely to be significant heterogeneity in the results
- B. A fixed-effect model is the least appropriate model for presenting the results
- C. In this scenario, a random-effect model should be used regardless of objective measures of heterogeneity
- D. No assessment of heterogeneity can be made
- E. The summary outcome on the Forest plot will inform us of heterogeneity

DOI: 10.1201/9781003221234-11

Q4. A new transplant maintenance drug has been used in a randomised controlled trial. Forty-five patients received the new maintenance drug, and 55 patients received the standard treatment. The 2-year transplant survival without rejection was 75% in the new drug group and 55% in the other. What would the number needed to treat be?

A. 10
B. 5
C. 55
D. 25
E. 45

Q5. A meta-analysis is performed comparing TACE with segmental hepatic resection. A total of six randomised controlled trials were included, and 5-year survival was seen to be greater in segmental hepatic resection. A funnel plot was used to assess publication bias, and an Egger test gave a p-value of 0.27. What is the most likely interpretation of publication bias?

A. There is no significant publication bias
B. There is significant publication bias
C. There is likely to be significant publication bias
D. There is unlikely to be significant publication bias
E. Publication bias can only be assessed adequately with an actual visual look at the funnel plot

Q6. A clinical question arises related to the benefits of using stents for metastatic oesophageal cancer versus palliative radiotherapy and you are tasked to produce a meta-analysis. During your literature search, you find two studies comparing stents versus palliative chemotherapy and one study comparing chemotherapy versus radiotherapy. What type of study would you perform?

A. Network meta-analysis
B. Conventional comparative meta-analysis
C. Diagnostic meta-analysis
D. Systematic review only
E. Scoping review

Q7. A prospective cohort study was performed investigating hospital stay in patients with appendicitis who were treated with oral or intravenous antibiotics. There were 55 patients in the oral antibiotic group and 60 in the intravenous group. There was no statistical significance between demographic groups. The median hospital stay in the oral antibiotic group was 5 days and that in the intravenous group was 3 days. What would be the best way to assess significance?

A. Wilcoxon test
B. Mann–Whitney U
C. Student T-test
D. Z-test
E. Fisher's exact test

Q8. An observational study was performed to determine the utility of Hartmann's intravenous fluid in the management of pancreatitis. Hospital stay was used as a primary end point, and a total of 322 patients were recruited with a Glasgow score of 2 or higher. The mean hospital stay was 4 days with a standard deviation of 2. When presenting your study, someone from the audience asks what the standard error of the mean would be.
A. 0.5
B. 4
C. 2
D. 36
E. 0.1

Q9. A national screening programme is organised in a Middle-Eastern country to identify breast cancers. After 10 years, the survival from ductal cancers was seen to have dramatically improved. What is the most likely reason for this?
A. Selection bias
B. Lead-time bias
C. Confirmation bias
D. Spectrum bias
E. Centripetal bias

Q10. A study is designed to investigate whether there is any difference in post-operative recovery between laparoscopic and robotic gastric bypass for obesity. There were 20 patients in the laparoscopic group and 22 patients in the robotic group. Hospital stay was seen to be 3 days in the robotic group and 7 days in the laparoscopic group. This difference was statistically significant and the first study to show this. Five studies from other centres previously failed to show this difference. How would you explain the results of your study?
A. Results from a centre of excellence
B. Differences related to the learning curve
C. Type I error
D. Type II error
E. False negatives

ANSWERS

Q1. Option A – 70%.
    The index test here is the CT scan with colonoscopy being the gold standard. The calculation for sensitivity is true positives divided by true positives plus false negatives. In this circumstance, the true positive value is 7 which was identified by both colonoscopy and CT and the false negatives are 3. Therefore, the sensitivity is 7 ÷ 10 which is 70%.

Q2. Option B – 11.
    The key here is to remember the principles of sensitivity and specificity. The gold standard is MRCP, and the sample size is 50. If 60% have stones on MRCP, then the number of positive stone patients is 30. The calculation we need is the positive predictive value because it is those that are false positives

TABLE 11.1

	MRCP Y	MRCP N
IOUSS Y	26 (TP)	11 (FP)
IOUSS N	4 (FN)	9 (TN)

Abbreviation: IOUSS, intraoperative ultrasound scan.

who will undergo an unnecessary cholangiogram. Working backwards, using the value of 26 patients as those who are true positive (26/30) using the sensitivity equation (true positives/true positives + false negatives) using 26 as the value, you get 26/37 as the positive predictive value. This gives 11 as the value for false-positive patients (Table 11.1).

Q3. Option C – In this scenario, a random-effect model should be used regardless of the objective measures of heterogeneity.

The assessment of whether to use fixed or random effects should be based on *a priori* information. There is already likely to be significant heterogeneity, and certainly, this is corroborated by the p-values being significant when comparing the demographic data. There is an argument not to even perform a summative analysis given the degree of discrepancy in demographic data. A random-effect model should be used (if a summative outcome is deemed appropriate) regardless of the objective measure (Chi(Q)) or IB because there are sufficient clinical differences to assume heterogeneity (or the old criticism of comparing apples with oranges!)

Q4. Option B – 5. The number needed to treat is calculated based on an absolute risk reduction. The exact calculation is the inverse of the ARR value. In this case, in the new drug group, there is a 25% risk of rejection; in the conventional group, there is 45%. The absolute risk reduction is 20% or 0.2. The inverse of this is 1/0.2, which equals 5. Note that the larger the risk reduction, the smaller the number needed to treat is.

Q5. Option C – There is likely to be significant publication bias.

Publication bias is generally assessed using a combination of a funnel plot and the Egger test. There are other tests that can be used to assess the significance of publication bias. If the Egger test is less than 0.05 (and in some studies, 0.1 is a more stringent test), then publication bias is considered significant. Interpreting funnel plots is more of a subjective assessment and looks at whether there is symmetry across a midpoint line. It should also follow the outer boundaries of the funnel plot to ensure that it does not fall outside these parameters. Appropriate assessment of publication bias based on these tools (Funnel plots and Egger tests) is usually only reliable when there are greater than ten studies included in the meta-analysis, and therefore, these tests cannot be interpreted. In this scenario, given that there are fewer than ten studies, there is inherently likely to be significant publication bias.

Q6. Option D – Systematic review only.

In this circumstance, there are no direct comparative studies which means that it is not possible to perform a conventional comparative meta-analysis. A diagnostic meta-analysis would be inappropriate given that these are interventions rather than investigations. When no direct comparative studies exist, a network analysis may be performed. This is based on having a common comparator with two interventions; i.e. you may have studies comparing A vs B and C vs B; using B as a common comparator, a comparison of A vs C may be conducted. In this case, there would be insufficient numbers of studies to perform even a comparative meta-analysis and so a network meta-analysis would be equally unachievable. Usually, four studies are considered good practice for conventional meta-analyses but they can be done with two studies. A scoping review is a type of literature review based on a topic. A mapping review is a type of literature review based on a question.

Q7. Option B – Mann–Whitney U.

In this case, given the use of median hospital stays, it implies a non-parametric distribution. A mean is more likely to represent a normal distribution and allows for parametric tests. Hospital stay is also a continuous data variable. The other aspect is whether the data is from a single sample or two independent samples. Given this, a Mann–Whitney U test would be the most appropriate test. If this was a single sample in the case of pain scores before or after intervention and considered as non-parametric data, a Wilcoxon test is used. A z-test is used when the variances are known, and a student t-test is performed when the variances are unknown (a more common scenario). Both of these tests are used in the context of a normal distribution. Fisher's exact test is used in non-continuous data and is useful for analyses where smaller sample sizes exist. A chi-squared test (which is more well-known) is the test used for samples that are larger.

Q8. Option E – 0.1.

There is great confusion between standard error and standard deviation. It is important to understand from the outset that these are two completely different statistics on two different sample sets. If you have one sample of results on 50 patients, a mean and standard deviation is reported on this single set of results. This sample of 50 patients, however, is a representative sample of the total population; e.g., you may look at hospital stay in 50 patients with pancreatitis, but in the world, there are many thousands of patients with pancreatitis. Therefore, 50 patients with pancreatitis are simply a sample. To offset this and to try and find a true mean value of the thousands of pancreatic patients, a number of studies of 50 or 60 or 100 patients are performed to get a better estimate. Each of the individual means of the study with 50, 60 or 100 patients will be slightly different and vary. These differences are what is being measured using the standard error (aka standard error of the mean). The standard error can also be calculated by the standard deviation and sample size of a particular study. This is done by the following: standard deviation/ $\sqrt{\text{sample size}}$. In the example above the sample size is 322. The closest whole number as a square root is 18 ($18 \times 18 = 324$). The standard error would therefore be $2/18 = 1/9 = 0.1$ (recurring).

Q9. Option B – Lead-time bias.

The lead-time bias is a general rule, especially when discussing screening. The lead-time bias is where a disease is picked up at an earlier point of the disease process and thus seemingly the period of survival is longer because it includes the period before a disease would have been diagnosed had it not been picked up by the screening process. Selection bias is where the study is performed on a group of patients that may not be reflective of the group of patients that are going to be treated. An example of this would be the treatment of obesity with exercise alone in patients who are highly motivated versus those that are not. Confirmation bias is where information is used to confirm or refute a hypothesis based upon pre-conceptions or what the investigator wants the result to be. Spectrum bias occurs mainly when diagnostic tests are involved and is where the environment in which the tests are used inevitably results in different groups of patients with different demographics. This is particularly seen in primary versus secondary or tertiary-care centres where there are more unwell patients in the secondary-/tertiary-care setting. Centripetal bias is where the number of cases in a particular centre may not reflect the whole region or country as patients may tend towards particular centres of excellence.

There is a good website that lists all types of bias and is well worth examining prior to the exam: https://catalogofbias.org/biases/selection-bias/

Q10. Option C – type I error.

The findings from the study essentially show a type I error which can also be defined as a false-positive finding. This study is at odds with the other studies and the likely true result is that there is no difference in hospital stay between the two techniques. In this circumstance, the results have falsely rejected the null hypothesis. A type II error is when the study inaccurately fails to reject the null hypothesis. The power of a study helps reduce the risk of a type II error. Although technically sample size should not affect a type I error, it is likely to be the cause for the type I error in this circumstance, given the discrepancy between the other studies. Type I errors are essentially defined by the significance level, so assuming your study design is accurate, the risk of type I error should not be affected by the sample size. In this scenario, more accurately, the type of error is a type III error where there has been model mis-specification or choosing a sample size or demographic that is not truly reflective of real life. The other options are of course possibilities, but given the number of studies going against your findings, a type I error is the most likely.

12 Transplant Surgery

Kiran Sran, Petrut Gogalniceanu, and Kaushal Kundalia

Q1. Which of the following organ donors are unlikely to be considered for solid organ donation after brain-stem death?
A. A 50-year-old man with a history of hepatitis C infection who had previously received direct acting antiviral (DAA) treatment. The donor was found to be HCV Ab-positive and HCV RNA negative at the time of potential donation.
B. A 50-year-old man with positive blood cultures for *Candida* on the day of the potential donation.
C. A 50-year-old woman with culture-proven bacterial meningitis, with an appropriate clinical response to antibiotic therapy by the time of potential donation.
D. A 50-year-old woman known to be HIV-positive, on highly active anti-retroviral therapy (HAART) with negative HIV RNA at the time of potential donation.
E. A 50-year-old man was found to be IgG-positive for *Toxoplasma gondii* at the time of potential donation.

Q2. Which of the following organ donors are unlikely to be considered for solid organ donation after brain-stem death?
A. A 65-year-old man who is 6 years post radical prostatectomy for Gleason 6 adenocarcinoma of the prostate, with undetectable PSA levels on annual follow-up
B. A 65-year-old man who underwent excision of a basal cell skin carcinoma 2 months prior to donation
C. A 45-year-old man undergoing radiotherapy for primary cerebral lymphoma
D. A 65-year-old woman who is over 10 years post curative surgery for a pT1 1.5 cm invasive breast cancer, with a negative mammogram 1 year prior to donation
E. A 45-year-old man who underwent partial left nephrectomy 6 months prior to donation for a 1 cm solitary renal cell carcinoma, Fuhrman grade 2

Q3. Mrs K, a 55-year-old woman with autosomal dominant polycystic kidney disease (ADPKD) is approaching end-stage renal failure. She has no living kidney donor options in her family. Her 60-year-old neighbour has come forward as a potential kidney donor, but the pair are ABO-incompatible. What is the best option for Mrs K moving forward, with regard to long-term renal replacement therapy?
A. Desensitisation and antibody removal prior to a direct living-donor kidney transplant from her neighbour
B. Activation on the deceased donor waiting list for kidney transplantation
C. Unit haemodialysis
D. Registration in a kidney sharing scheme for living-donor kidney transplantation
E. Home haemodialysis

DOI: 10.1201/9781003221234-12

Q4. Mr D is a 50-year-old gentleman with IgA nephropathy, who is rapidly approaching end-stage renal failure. He has had a previous open appendicectomy and left inguinal hernia repair. He is keen to continue working full-time as a lawyer. He has good calibre vessels in both his arm. His wife is a compatible living kidney donor, but it will take several months before the pair will be ready to proceed with elective surgery. Which of the following is the most appropriate next step in Mr D's management?

A. Formation of a radiocephalic AV fistula in preparation for home haemodialysis.

B. Formation of a radiocephalic AV fistula in preparation for unit haemodialysis.

C. Insertion of a tunnelled haemodialysis catheter when the commencement of dialysis is indicated.

D. Insertion of a temporary haemodialysis catheter when the commencement of dialysis is indicated.

E. Insertion of a peritoneal dialysis catheter.

Q5. A 12-year-old girl with focal segmental glomerulosclerosis undergoes renal transplantation from a blood group and HLA-compatible living donor. Post-transplantation, her serum creatinine fell consistently until day 4, when significant lower limb oedema, ascites and proteinuria were noted, along with a rise in serum creatinine. A biopsy of the allograft was performed urgently. What is the most likely diagnosis?

A. Acute antibody-mediated rejection

B. Calcineurin inhibitor toxicity

C. Recurrence of focal segmental glomerulosclerosis

D. Post-transplant lymphoproliferative disorder

E. BK nephropathy

Q6. Which of the following patients with end-stage renal failure are suitable for immediate activation on the deceased donor waiting list for renal transplantation?

A. A 55-year-old woman with polycystic kidney disease who has had three admissions to the hospital in the last 6 months with fever and right-sided flank pain

B. A 60-year-old man who had bilateral native nephrectomies for pT3 renal cell carcinoma 2 years ago

C. A 65-year-old man who underwent cystectomy with ileal conduit formation for multifocal superficial bladder cancer 8 years ago

D. A 35-year-old woman with IgA nephropathy whose first kidney transplant is failing, with an eGFR of 16 mL/min

E. A 60-year-old man with hypertensive nephropathy and AF, who is on Apixaban 2.5 mg bd

Q7. A 30-year-old man develops ipsilateral leg swelling 2 weeks following deceased donor kidney transplantation and swelling in the right iliac fossa at the site of the allograft. His serum creatinine is unchanged at 90–100 μmol/L. Doppler scanning excludes lower limb deep-vein thrombosis. What is the most likely cause?

A. Renal vein thrombosis

B. Urine leak

    C. Lymphocoele
    D. Ureteric stenosis
    E. Renal artery stenosis

Q8. A 45-year-old man undergoes routine ureteric stent removal 4 weeks after deceased donor renal transplantation. Over the following days, his urine output declines, serum creatinine begins to rise and he experiences discomfort over the allograft. What is the most likely cause?
    A. Lymphocoele
    B. Renal artery thrombosis
    C. Renal vein thrombosis
    D. Ureteric stenosis
    E. Renal artery stenosis

Q9. Which of the following is not a common indication of allograft nephrectomy?
    A. Early renal vein thrombosis
    B. Space for re-transplantation
    C. Anaemia resistant to treatment
    D. Post-transplant lymphoproliferative disorder
    E. Chronic pyelonephritis

Q10. Which of the following insulin-treated diabetic patients are eligible to be immediately listed for the simultaneous pancreas and kidney transplantation?
    A. A 35-year-old man with type 2 diabetes and a calculated GFR of 22 mL/min, with a BMI of 23 kg/m^2
    B. A 35-year-old man with type 1 diabetes and a calculated GFR of 22 mL/min, with a BMI of 23 kg/m^2
    C. A 35-year-old woman with type 2 diabetes on haemodialysis, with a BMI of 31 kg/m^2
    D. A 35-year-old man with type 2 diabetes and a calculated GFR of 15 mL/min, with a BMI of 31 kg/m^2
    E. A 35-year-old woman with type 1 diabetes on peritoneal dialysis, with a BMI of 23 kg/m^2

Q11. A 65-year-old woman on long-term haemodialysis presents with progressive tachycardia, tachypnoea, elevated JVP and peripheral oedema. She has a right brachiocephalic AV fistula with a flow rate of 2.5 L/min, two areas of moderate aneurysmal dilatation as well as US evidence of several 50%–75% stenoses within the fistula vein. Dialysis parameters and adequacy are within normal limits. Which of the following interventions are not indicated?
    A. Revision of the brachiocephalic fistula with an interposition PTFE graft
    B. Percutaneous fistuloplasty of the flow-limiting stenoses
    C. Ligation of the brachiocephalic fistula and placement of a permanent tunnelled catheter for haemodialysis
    D. Flow reduction procedure
    E. Ligation of the brachiocephalic fistula and placement of a brachioaxillary PTFE arteriovenous graft

Q12. A 30-year-old man with polycystic kidney disease is assessed in your clinic with a view to arteriovenous fistula formation. His current eGFR is 12 and he is right-handed. The mapping of his upper limb veins is as follows:

Right Arm		Left Arm	
CV at wrist	3 mm	CV at wrist	1.8 mm
RA at wrist	2.5 mm	RA at wrist	2.2 mm
CV at ACF	4.2 mm	CV at ACF	2.4 mm
BV at ACF	4.5 mm	BV at ACF	4.8 mm
BA at ACF	4 mm	BA at ACF	4 mm

Bilateral axillary and subclavian veins are noted to be patent. Which of the following is your most preferred option for vascular access?
A. Left radiocephalic AV fistula
B. Right radiocephalic AV fistula
C. Left brachiobasilic AV fistula
D. Right brachiocephalic AV fistula
E. Left brachioaxillary AV graft

Q13. In pancreatic whole-organ transplantation, which of the following combinations of donor and recipient arteries are most commonly used to facilitate arterial supply to the allograft?
A. Donor: superior mesenteric, splenic and external, internal and common iliac arteries
   Recipient: aorta
B. Donor: coeliac trunk
   Recipient: aorta
C. Donor: superior mesenteric, splenic and external, internal and common iliac arteries
   Recipient: common iliac artery
D. Donor: coeliac trunk
   Recipient: common iliac artery
E. Donor: superior mesenteric, splenic and external, internal and common carotid arteries
   Recipient: common iliac artery

Q14. Which of the following is the most common anatomical variation seen, relevant to organ retrieval and liver transplantation?
A. Common hepatic artery originating directly from the aorta
B. Common hepatic artery arising from the superior mesenteric artery
C. Aberrant left hepatic artery arising from the superior mesenteric artery
D. Aberrant left hepatic artery arising from the left gastric artery
E. Aberrant right hepatic artery arising from the inferior mesenteric artery

Q15. Which of the following is the most common anatomical variant seen, relevant to organ retrieval and renal transplantation?
   A. Unilateral renal agenesis
   B. Horseshoe kidney
   C. Crossed ectopic kidney
   D. Pelvic kidney
   E. Intrathoracic kidney

Q16. A 65-year-old man underwent kidney transplantation 15 years ago. He presents with abdominal pain, distension and vomiting. A CT scan shows widespread abdominal lymphadenopathy. Serum LDH is elevated. Which of the following viruses is likely to be responsible for this pathology?
   A. CMV
   B. HTLV
   C. EBV
   D. Coronavirus
   E. Hepatitis E

Q17. A 76-year-old right-handed female attends the clinic for the formation of permanent vascular access for haemodialysis. She has had heavy cannulation of the cephalic vein in the left forearm. The cephalic vein above the elbow is very small. Which of the following veins should be the primary target vascular access formation, provided the patient has no preference?
   A. Left brachial veins
   B. Left basilic vein
   C. Right cephalic vein at the antecubital fossa
   D. Left axillary vein
   E. Right internal jugular vein

Q18. A 75-year-old female has undergone dialysis via a right brachiocephalic AV fistula for the last 7 years. She weighs 68 kg. An ultrasound duplex scan suggests a flow rate of 450 mL/min with a post-anastomotic stenosis of 70%. What is the best form of intervention?
   A. Proximalisation of the cephalic vein
   B. Insertion of an interposition graft
   C. Surgical revision of the anastomosis and on-table sequential dilatation of the lesion
   D. Endovascular balloon angioplasty in interventional radiology
   E. Conservative management in light of flow rates and age of fistula.

Q19. A 79-year-old male with long-standing diabetes has a left brachiocephalic AV fistula formed under local anaesthesia. Three weeks later he presents to the clinic with recurrent pain in the left hand whenever he performs light work in the garden. On examination, the hand is cool and mildly dusky with thickened skin in the digital tips. What is the likely cause of this?
   A. Brachial artery stenosis with poor run-off in the left hand
   B. Intra-operative nerve damage leading to neuropathic pain
   C. Venous hypertension secondary to proximal central venous stenosis
   D. Steal syndrome from the AV fistula
   E. Carpal tunnel syndrome

Q20. A 69-year-old woman presents with pain in the left hand where she has a brachiocephalic AV fistula. The pain is worse on dialysis. The hand is cold with thenar wasting and fingertip infarcts. An US duplex scan shows flow rates of 3,000 mL/min. Which of the following is not a recognised treatment option?
   A. Fistula ligation
   B. Banding of the fistula inflow
   C. DRIL procedure (distal revascularisation, interval ligation)
   D. Balloon angioplasty and stenting of the AV fistula anastomosis
   E. RUDI procedure (revision using distal inflow)

Q21. A 25-year-old male undergoes a living-donor transplant from his father. He receives induction with Basiliximab and is maintained on triple immunosuppression therapy in the form of tacrolimus, mycophenolate mofetil and prednisolone. Three weeks later, he represents with loose stool. The dose of which of the following immunosuppression agents will need adjustment?
   A. Mycophenolate mofetil
   B. Tacrolimus
   C. Prednisolone
   D. Sirolimus
   E. Cyclosporin

Q22. A 38-year-old female undergoes a deceased donor kidney transplant. The donor's kidney arrives with a retrieval injury consisting of a very short ureter. This cannot reach the recipient's bladder. Which of the following is not a recognised method of rescuing this situation?
   A. Boari flap
   B. Ureteric anastomosis to native ipsilateral ureter
   C. Cutaneous ureterostomy
   D. MILLER procedure
   E. Bladder hitch

Q23. A 19-year-old male has end-stage renal failure secondary to IgA nephropathy. He receives a living-donor kidney from his mother, with evidence of urine production on the table from the reperfused allograft. In recovery, the patient suddenly stops passing urine. His blood pressure is 150/88 mmHg. The nurse has already flushed the catheter and bladder scanning confirms an empty bladder. A 500 mL fluid bolus has no effect on urine output. What do you do next?
   A. Take the patient back to the theatre and re-explore immediately
   B. CT angiogram to look for transplant renal artery stenosis (TRAS)
   C. US duplex of the kidney to exclude renal vein thrombosis
   D. US-guided renal biopsy to diagnose early recurrence of IgA nephropathy
   E. Check donor-specific antibodies (DSA) in case the patient is having acute rejection

Q24. A 45-year-old female undergoes renal transplantation from a DBD donor. Her drain output is 600 mL of clear yellow fluid per day on day 3 following surgery. Her serum creatinine has fallen to 125. Her drain fluid creatinine is >500. What is the most appropriate next treatment option?
   A. Flexible cystoscopy and stent removal
   B. Consideration of surgical re-exploration and ureteric reimplantation

C. Removal of the drain and repeat US scan in 1 week
D. CT of the abdomen and pelvis with contrast (urographic phase)
E. Urinary diversion by means of percutaneous nephrostomy

Q25. A 65-year-old renal transplant patient with diabetes presents with cloudy urine, dysuria and pain over the transplanted kidney. Urinalysis is positive for leucocytes and nitrites. He has a temperature of 38.4°C, a heart rate of 110 and a blood pressure of 123/89 mmHg. He is on tacrolimus, mycophenolate mofetil (MMF) and prednisolone. Which of the following changes will you make to his immunosuppression therapy?
   A. Stop all immunosuppression medications
   B. Continue all medications, but speak to the transplant nephrologist in the morning when they are back at work in order to get tertiary advice
   C. Stop MMF, reduce the tacrolimus dose and double the prednisolone dose
   D. Stop the tacrolimus, reduce the MMF and double the prednisolone dose
   E. Stop the tacrolimus, reduce the MMF and half the prednisolone dose

Q26. A 32-year male presents to A&E with sudden onset but mild pain in the right iliac fossa. He is noted to have had a previous simultaneous pancreas and kidney transplant, together with appendicectomy. This was noted to have been complicated by an enteric leak at the time. Currently, he has ongoing moderate pain. His blood pressure is 120/86 mmHg with a heart rate of 86 beats/minute. His serum glucose level is 6. His serum amylase is 24. He is passing good volumes of urine, and his creatinine is at the baseline. How would you manage this next?
   A. HbA1C levels and C-peptide levels
   B. Donor-specific antibodies
   C. US scan in the morning
   D. CT angiogram immediately
   E. Non-contrast CT scan of the abdomen to avoid renal injury

Q27. A 26-year-old female with a previous deceased donor kidney transplant presents with a rise in creatinine over several weeks. An ultrasound of her renal transplant shows moderately raised resistive indices but is otherwise unremarkable. Percutaneous allograft biopsy shows antibody-mediated rejection. Which of the following is a therapeutic option?
   A. Plasma exchange
   B. ATG (anti-thymocyte globulin)
   C. ACE inhibitor
   D. Tranexamic acid
   E. Urgent re-transplantation using a living donor

Q28. A 45-year-old male undergoes an uneventful laparoscopic living-donor left nephrectomy, to donate to his 4-year-old son. He returns to the clinic 3 weeks later with left-sided scrotal pain. What is the most likely diagnosis?
   A. Damage to the pre-sacral nerve plexus
   B. Urine leak from the ureteric stump, tracking to his scrotum
   C. Varicocoele
   D. Inguino-scrotal hernia
   E. Hydrocoele

Q29. A 41-year-old male suffers a sub-arachnoid haemorrhage, and brain-stem death is confirmed. He is on the organ donor register. Which of the following donor factors should concern the implanting surgeon most with respect to deceased donor kidney transplantation?
   A. High alcohol consumption
   B. A history of skin squamous cell carcinoma 6 years ago which underwent a curative resection
   C. Previous cytomegalovirus (CMV) infection
   D. Previous epstein-Barr virus (EBV) infection
   E. Hypertension on three anti-hypertensive agents

Q30. A 68-year-old male has been on peritoneal dialysis for 6 years. He presents with abdominal pain, distension, vomiting and complete constipation. The PD fluid is clear. A CT scan of his abdomen and pelvis shows small bowel obstruction with no evidence of herniation, lymphadenopathy, organomegaly or malignancy. How do you manage this condition?
   A. Immediate laparotomy and formation of defunctioning ileostomy
   B. NG drainage, total parenteral nutrition and referral to a specialist unit
   C. Intra-peritoneal antibiotics via a PD catheter
   D. Commence rituximab and CHOP chemotherapy
   E. Removal of PD tube and resting of the peritoneal membrane for 2 weeks, prior to re-attempting peritoneal dialysis

Q31. What is the UKELD cut-off for listing chronic liver disease patients for liver transplantation in the UK?
   A. <48
   B. ≤48
   C. =49
   D. >49
   E. ≥49

Q32. Which of the following is one of the variables used to calculate the UKELD score?
   A. Serum chloride
   B. Serum magnesium
   C. Serum sodium
   D. Serum potassium
   E. Serum calcium

Q33. Which of the following is/are indications for liver transplantation?
   A. Nodular regenerative hyperplasia with portal hypertension not responding to medical/endoscopic management
   B. Unresectable hepatoblastoma
   C. Hepatocellular carcinoma (single 4 cm lesion) in child C cirrhosis liver
   D. B and C
   E. All of the above

Q34. Which of the following is a de-selection criterion for liver transplantation?
   A. Porto-pulmonary hypertension not responding to medical management
   B. Hepatopulmonary syndrome in the absence of chronic lung disease
   C. Recurrent skin infections secondary to intractable pruritus
   D. Nodular regenerative hyperplasia
   E. Chronic hepatic encephalopathy

Q35. A 56-year-old male patient underwent deceased donor liver transplantation for primary sclerosing cholangitis (PSC). A few hours after the transplant, the intensivist is concerned about increasing inotropic support, high haemorrhagic drain output, worsening LFTs and coagulation profile. What should be the next step in management?
   A. Immediate re-exploration
   B. CT abdomen with contrast
   C. Correction of coagulopathy
   D. Continue conservative management in ITU
   E. Liver Biopsy

Q36. During abdominal organ retrieval from a donor with brain-stem death, the retrieval surgeon notes a severely calcified infra-renal aorta. Which of the following alternative sites can be used for aortic cannulation?
   A. Right common iliac artery
   B. Left common iliac artery
   C. Left external Iiiac artery
   D. Antegrade thoracic aortic cannulation
   E. All of the above

Q37. A 56-year-old male patient underwent a DCD liver transplant with duct-to-duct biliary reconstruction, for NASH. Two years post-transplant, the patient presented with cholangitis. On further investigations, a biliary stricture in proximal CBD was noted, extending up to just below the biliary confluence. What would be the next step in management?
   A. ERCP and stenting
   B. Percutaneous transhepatic biliary drainage (PTBD) and stenting
   C. Surgical revision of biliary reconstruction
   D. Re-listing for liver transplant
   E. Step-up immunosuppressive drug regime

Q38. A 56-year-old male patient underwent a deceased donor liver transplant with Roux-en-y biliary reconstruction, for NASH. Two years post-transplant, the patient re-presents with cholangitis. On further investigations, a biliary stricture in proximal CBD was noted, extending to just below the biliary confluence. What would be the next step in management?
   A. ERCP and stenting
   B. PTBD and stenting
   C. Surgical revision of biliary reconstruction
   D. Re-listing for liver transplant
   E. Step-up immunosuppressive drug regime

Q39. Which of the following is not true regarding liver transplants?
- A. Calculous cholecystitis is a common cause of biliary sepsis after a liver transplant
- B. Non-anastomotic biliary strictures are commonly related to ischaemia of biliary epithelium
- C. Management of primary non-function is a super-urgent listing for a second liver transplant on an emergency basis
- D. Ischaemic cholangiopathy is more common with DCD liver transplants than with DBD liver transplants
- E. DCD liver transplants have a better outcome when the WIT < 20 minutes and the CIT < 8 hours

ANSWERS

Q1. Option B – A 50-year-old man with positive blood cultures for *Candida* on the day of the potential donation.

The benefits of a deceased donor solid organ transplant should be balanced with the potential risks of infection transmission between donor and recipient, particularly in the context of post-transplant immunosuppression.

Absolute contraindications to solid organ donation include:
- CJD
- Untreated bacteriaemia or fungaemia
- Viral meningoencephalitis

Donation is permissible in the case of:
- Hepatitis B or C, HIV or HTLV infection
- CMV or EBV infection
- *Toxoplasma gondii*

The decision to proceed with solid organ transplantation in this context depends on a careful assessment of the risk versus benefit, with appropriate counselling of the potential transplant recipient as well as appropriate post-transplant monitoring.

Q2. Option B – A 65-year-old man who underwent excision of a basal cell skin carcinoma 2 months prior to donation

Organs from deceased donors with certain types of current and past cancers may be safely used for transplantation. The risks of cancer transmission must be balanced against the risks of the patient dying while waiting for a transplant, and the patient must be appropriately counselled and must give informed consent.

In the context of past or current donor cancers, absolute contraindications for solid organ transplant include:
- Primary cerebral lymphoma
- All secondary intracranial tumours
- Active haematological malignancy
- Cancers with metastatic spread

The risk of disease transmission varies with the type of cancer, treatment and disease-free period in the donor. This risk is perceived to be low to minimal with certain types of CNS, kidney, prostate, thyroid and skin cancers.

Q3. Option D – Registration in a kidney sharing scheme for living-donor kidney transplantation.

Kidney transplantation from a living donor, when available, is the treatment of choice for most patients with end-stage renal failure, offering optimum patient and graft survival, and reduced time on the national waiting list.

The UK Living Kidney Sharing Scheme is one of the most successful in Europe and enables donor-recipient pairs, who are HLA or ABO-incompatible, to achieve compatible transplants with other similar pairs in the country.

A successful match in the scheme is likely to confer the following benefits:
• A shorter waiting time for a transplant as compared to the deceased donor programme
• A better quality of life and increased life expectancy as compared to long-term dialysis
• Better outcomes and increased graft and patient survival as compared to deceased donor transplant, or antibody removal treatment prior to an incompatible living-donor kidney transplant

Q4. Option E – Insertion of a peritoneal dialysis catheter.

The decision for peritoneal dialysis vs haemodialysis is coloured by multiple factors including patient age, motivation, geographic distance from a HD unit, and transplantation prospects.

Some of the benefits of peritoneal dialysis over haemodialysis include:
• Better preservation of residual kidney function
• Better preservation of urine output in preparation for transplantation
• Better ability to maintain daily activities including work and travel
• Reduced exposure to the hospital environment and hospital-acquired infections
In the case of the patient described above, who has a potential living donor in work-up, both short-term haemodialysis via a tunnelled catheter and peritoneal dialysis are reasonable options for renal replacement therapy as a bridge to transplantation.

With particular reference to the patient's age and work schedule, PD is likely to offer him the advantages mentioned above. Previous appendicectomy and inguinal hernia repair are not contraindications to PD.

Fistula formation is not indicated in this case, where short-term dialysis prior to transplantation is anticipated.

Q5. Option C – Recurrence of FSGS

Focal segmental glomerulosclerosis (FSGS) is one of the most common causes of nephrotic syndrome in children, often leading to end-stage renal failure. The risk of recurrence of primary or idiopathic FSGS post-transplantation can be as high as 80% and may occur within hours to days of transplantation. Risk factors for recurrent FSGS include younger age at the onset of initial disease, rapid progression to ESRF, and loss of the previous allograft to recurrent disease.

The hallmark of recurrent FSGS is proteinuria, often diagnosed within days of transplantation, with the clinical picture of nephrotic syndrome. Treatment is most commonly with plasma exchange and rituximab.

Q6. Option C – A 65-year-old man who underwent cystectomy with ileal conduit formation for multifocal superficial bladder cancer 8 years ago.

A patient with ESRF and recurring urinary tract infections requiring hospital admission needs further investigation of the entire urinary tract prior to consideration of transplantation. This is likely to entail cross-sectional imaging, cystoscopy with or without ureteral barbotage, or urodynamic studies. With particular reference to patients with polycystic kidney disease, recurrent cyst infections may necessitate unilateral or bilateral native nephrectomy prior to transplantation.

An ileal conduit following curative surgery for superficial bladder cancer, with a disease-free period of over 8 years, is not a contraindication to kidney transplant. The implant procedure, however, will be technically challenging in view of the previous dissection for iliac lymphadenopathy, as well as the dilemma of how to manage the transplant ureter. In the context of deceased donor transplantation, cutaneous ureterostomy may be the best option.

A patient with chronic kidney disease can only be listed for deceased donor transplantation when their eGFR is consistently <15 mL/min.

Direct oral anticoagulant (DOAC) therapy is particularly challenging in the context of deceased donor transplantation due to the need for timely reversal and surgery, and the limited availability of an appropriate reversal agent. For the purposes of deceased donor listing, switching to an alternative anticoagulant such as warfarin is often recommended.

Q7. Option C – Lymphocoele

The development of a lymphocoele is a common complication after renal transplantation. They are usually asymptomatic, incidentally found on routine scanning of the allograft, and may resolve with time. Large lymphocoeles, however, can cause abdominal swelling or discomfort, and pressure effect on the hilum of the kidney allograft, iliac vessels and the transplant ureter. Consequences may include urinary frequency due to pressure on the bladder, ipsilateral leg swelling or deep-vein thrombosis due to iliac venous compression or transplant hydronephrosis causing graft dysfunction due to the compression of the ureter in the absence of a ureteric stent. This is most commonly managed with percutaneous drainage under image control. In the event of persistent drainage of large amounts of lymph, surgical fenestration into the peritoneal cavity may be indicated, which can be performed via open or laparoscopic approaches.

Q8. Option D – Ureteric stenosis

The indwelling ureteric stent, placed at the time of transplantation, is routinely removed at 4–6 weeks post-surgery. It is at this point that ureteric complications such as stenosis may become apparent. Ureteric obstruction usually manifests as graft dysfunction with evidence of worsening hydronephrosis on ultrasound. The management of this is with urgent percutaneous nephrostomy in the first instance, followed by a nephrostogram and antegrade stenting.

Depending on the length of the stricture, definitive surgical options include direct ureteric reimplantation to the bladder or anastomosis to the native ureter.

Q9. Option D – Post-transplant lymphoproliferative disorder

The indications for transplant nephrectomy in the early post-transplant period include graft thrombosis (arterial or venous), refractory acute rejection, overwhelming sepsis, post-biopsy bleeding, or primary non-function. In the later post-transplant period, indications include chronic rejection causing graft tenderness or persistent haematuria, anaemia, recurrent infections, or malignant tumours within the allograft. There may also be a need for graft nephrectomy as a preliminary measure in preparation for re-transplantation, e.g., for a third transplant or following combined organ transplantation.

The incidence of post-transplant lymphoproliferative disorder (PTLD) in kidney transplant recipients is approximately 2%. Presenting symptoms include fever, night sweats, weight loss and lymphadenopathy. Although PTD may involve the transplanted kidney, the mainstay of management is the reduction of immunosuppression and chemotherapy.

Q10. Option E – A 35-year-old woman with type 1 diabetes on peritoneal dialysis, with a BMI of 23 kg/m^2

Whole-organ pancreas transplantation is a viable treatment option for selected people with diabetes. Patients who develop end-stage renal failure secondary to either Type 1 or Type 2 diabetes, who are on insulin and are not obese may be considered for simultaneous pancreas-kidney transplantation. In the UK, the Pancreas Advisory Group has agreed on criteria to guide decisions on recipient selection, which include the following:
- All patients listed for pancreas transplantation should have insulin-treated diabetes
- Patients listed for simultaneous kidney–pancreas transplant must also be receiving dialysis or have a calculated/measured GFR of 20 mL/min or less at the time of listing
- Patients listed for pancreas transplantation with type 2 diabetes must have a calculated BMI of 30 kg/m^2 or less at the time of listing

Q11. Option B – Percutaneous fistuloplasty of the flow-limiting stenoses

The clinical picture presented is that of high-output cardiac failure secondary to an upper arm AV fistula with high volume flow. Coincidentally, there is also evidence of aneurysmal change and stenosis in the AV fistula, though dialysis remains adequate. The various management options for a high-flow AV fistula include inflow reduction by means of banding procedures or revision of the anastomosis, the use of an interposition graft to replace aneurysmal segments or ligation of the AV fistula and placement of alternative dialysis access.

In this case, fistuloplasty of the stenotic lesions is likely to result in an increase in flow within the fistula, thereby exacerbating cardiac failure.

Q12. Option B – Right radiocephalic AV fistula

The general principles underlying decision-making in vascular access formation include non-dominant arm over dominant, distal before proximal, native options before prosthetic, and upper limb before lower. As a rule of thumb, poor outcomes are observed with vein diameters <2 mm.

In the case of the above-described patient, the veins in his left arm are small on the mapping scan, with the exception of the basilic vein. The formation of a brachio-basilic AV fistula would often involve a two-stage procedure and is less preferable in a young patient with forearm options, albeit in his dominant arm. A brachiocephalic AV fistula remains an option, though the CV is noted to be of fairly small calibre and appropriate risk/benefit discussion with the patient needs to be undertaken.

On the right, the patient has excellent calibre veins and arteries in the forearm and upper arm, and he would benefit most from a right radiocephalic AV fistula, preserving his venous capital for the future.

Q13. Option C – Donor: superior mesenteric, splenic and external, internal and common iliac arteries; Recipient: common iliac artery

The pancreas allograft receives arterial inflow from two sources: the donor superior mesenteric artery, which supplies the head of the pancreas via the inferior pancreaticoduodenal artery, and the donor splenic artery, which supplies the body and the tail. The donor common, internal and external iliac arteries are also retrieved, which are anastomosed to the donor SMA and splenic arteries on the back-table to form a Y-graft, providing a single arterial inflow. This common iliac artery portion is then most commonly anastomosed to the recipient's common iliac artery.

The donor portal vein is the main graft vein, which drains the donor splenic and superior mesenteric veins. This is commonly anastomosed to the recipient IVC or common iliac vein.

The pancreas is retrieved with a segment of the donor duodenum, which is shortened on the back-table. Drainage of the exocrine secretions of the pancreas can be facilitated by anastomosis to the bladder or jejunum, though the latter is now the most common.

Q14. Option D – Aberrant left hepatic artery arising from the left gastric artery

The arterial supply to the liver varies significantly, with variations seen in approximately 40% of people. The classic anatomical pattern (seen in 60% of the population) is where the common hepatic artery arises from the coeliac trunk to form the gastroduodenal and proper hepatic arteries. The latter then divides into the right and left branches to supply the entire liver.

Aberrant arteries may be either replaced or accessory; replaced arteries arise are a substitute for the classical hepatic artery supply to a part of the liver, while an accessory artery is present in addition to an artery supplying that segment arising from a more standard anatomical position.

The most common variants are that of a replaced left hepatic artery arising from the left gastric artery (10%–15%) and replaced right hepatic artery arising from the superior mesenteric artery (10%–15%).

Q15. Option B – Horseshoe kidney

Horseshoe kidney is the most common renal malformation, with an incidence of approximately 1:400 to 600, and may be identified at the time of deceased donor organ retrieval. The vascular and ureteric anatomy is variable – the arterial supply may arise from iliac arteries, sacral arteries, mesenteric arteries as well as the aorta. The ureters pass anterior to the fused lower poles and run medially. The isthmus of the horseshoe is variable in size, and it may be possible to split the kidney in the case of a narrow isthmus, for use in two recipients. Alternatively, the whole horseshoe may be transplanted into 1 recipient *en bloc* using the donor aorta and IVC.

Q16. Option C – EBV

The Epstein-Barr virus can cause PTLD. This is a form of B-cell lymphoma presenting predominantly with fever, night sweats, weight loss and lymphadenopathy. It may be associated with raised serum LDH levels. PTLD localised to the small bowel can result in a bowel obstruction or perforation. Treatment involves a reduction in immunosuppression therapy and systemic chemotherapy.

Q17. Option C – Right cephalic vein at the antecubital fossa

The cephalic vein is the primary vein used in the formation of AV fistulas (AVFs), such as radiocephalic or brachio-cephalic fistulas. AVFs should be formed in the non-dominant arm to allow full use of the dominant upper limb during haemodialysis. Where the cephalic vein in the non-dominant arm is not an option for fistula formation, other options include the creation of a two-stage brachiobasilic fistula, insertion of a PTFE arteriovenous graft, formation of a fistula in the dominant limb. Patient preference plays a large role in the decision-making process. In this particular case, a brachiocephalic fistula in the dominant arm is most likely to be the right choice.

Q18. Option D – Endovascular balloon angioplasty in interventional radiology

The flow in a brachiocephalic AV fistula should ideally be over 800 mL/min. Low flow rates are associated with inadequate dialysis and eventual thrombosis with loss of dialysis access. High-grade stenoses that are flow-limiting should be treated by endovascular means in the first instance if possible. With a poor inflow as in this case, an interposition PTFE graft would not be a suitable option. Surgical revision should be considered when endovascular therapy fails.

Q19. Option D – Steal syndrome from the AV fistula

Steal syndrome occurs when AV fistulas are formed and the resultant high flow creates relative ischaemia in the hand. This can be exacerbated by exercise or during dialysis. Similarly, it may occur in patients with diabetes that have microvascular disease in the hand or heavily calcific disease in the radial and ulnar arteries. This often presents with a cool, dusky and painful hand. Doppler ultrasonography may reveal a high-flow AV fistula with a reversal of flow in the artery distal to the anastomosis. Symptoms may be relieved by temporary compression of the fistula.

New AVF formation can also cause hand swelling, which in turn may exacerbate subclinical carpal tunnel syndrome. This is an important differential diagnosis which can be made with the aid of nerve conduction studies.

Q20. Option D – Balloon angioplasty and stenting of the AV fistula anastomosis

Ischaemic symptoms or tissue loss in the hand distal to an AV fistula requires surgical intervention. Options include revision (DRIL or RUDI procedure), inflow reduction of the fistula (banding) or ligation. The purpose of the intervention is to reduce flow in the fistula. Angioplasty of the AV anastomosis would have the opposite effect.

Q21. Option A – Mycophenolate mofetil

Mycophenolate mofetil (MMF) is the principal cause of loose stools in transplant recipients. Cyclosporin is associated with hirsutism and gingival hypertrophy. Tacrolimus is nephrotoxic, neurotoxic (commonly causing tremors), and is associated with new-onset diabetes after transplantation (NODAT). Sirolimus is associated with impaired wound healing and should be replaced prior to elective surgery in transplant patients.

Q22. Option D – MILLER procedure

A MILLER procedure (minimally invasive limited ligation endoluminal-assisted revision) is a surgical approach in the management of steal syndrome associated with vascular access for haemodialysis. The remaining options allow drainage of a transplanted kidney with a short ureter. With a cutaneous ureterostomy, the ureter of the donor's kidney is brought out to the skin with drainage of urine into a bag. Alternatively, the ureter can be anastomosed to the recipient's native ureter on the same side. With a bladder hitch, the bladder is mobilised and moved closer to the renal pelvis. In a Boari flap, a segment of the bladder is tubularised and used as a conduit on which the ureter can be anastomosed.

Q23. Option A – Take the patient back to the theatre and re-explore immediately

A sudden drop or cessation in urine output following a renal transplant should always be treated as a vascular emergency. The most likely causes are renal vein thrombosis or renal artery thrombosis. These are often early complications related to surgical technique. Surgeons should not hesitate to re-explore quickly.

Q24. Option E – Urinary diversion by means of percutaneous nephrostomy

This patient has a urine leak as suggested by a disproportionately high drain fluid creatinine level as compared to that of serum. Urine leaks may occur at the level of the bladder, ureter or renal calyx, though are most likely as a result of a non-water-tight neoureterocystostomy or bladder closure. The initial management involves the immediate placement of a urinary catheter (if this has already been removed) to reduce intravesical pressure. This may reduce or stop leakage altogether. However, when leaks occur early, surgical exploration and repair are usually required. If the ureteric leak is a simple anastomotic leak, resection of the distal ureter and reimplantation is the easiest. However, if the ureter is non-viable because of inadequate blood supply, anastomosis of the renal pelvis to the native ureter is a good option. Percutaneous treatment may be difficult when there is no hydronephrosis or dilatation of the collecting system.

Q25. Option C – Stop MMF, reduce the tacrolimus dose and double the prednisolone dose

Immunosuppression advice should always be sought from a transplant centre nephrologist on a 24-hour basis. Should this not be possible, in a patient with sepsis, the MMF should be reduced or stopped, the tacrolimus dose reduced and the steroid dose increased so as to compensate for the stress response.

Q26. Option D – CT angiogram immediately

Vascular anastomoses in pancreas transplants are susceptible to pseudoaneurysm formation. These are caused by peri-pancreatic secretions in the immediate post-operative setting. In this case, the presence of enteric content increases the risks of an infective pseudoaneurysm. These can be potentially life-threatening in the event of a rupture. The absence of severe pain or shock should not be reassuring, as pain can be a sentinel presentation prior to rupture. Initial management involves CT angiography and the potential deployment of a covered stent over the Y-graft origin. Non-contrast scans are not diagnostic and the use of contrast can be justified in such cases.

Q27. Option A – Plasma exchange

Plasma exchange allows the removal of antibodies and can be used in conjunction with intravenous immunoglobulin (IVIG). Plasma exchange also removes albumin and clotting factors, leading to coagulopathy. This may require the replacement of blood products. ATG is usually used in cellular-mediated rejection.

Q28. Option C – Varicoele

Removal of the left kidney involves ligation of the left gonadal vein. In a small proportion of men, this can manifest as left scrotal discomfort, as a result of venous congestion. This may result in a varicocoele. Initial management is conservative with scrotal support. Referral to a urological surgeon is advised if symptoms do not settle.

Q29. Option E – Hypertension on three anti-hypertensive agents

CMV and EBV viral infections are relevant for recipient follow-up but are not contraindications to transplantation. Similarly, high alcohol consumption in the absence of hepato-renal syndrome is an acceptable risk factor. A previous history of cancer more than 5 years prior to donation is not a contraindication to the donation provided the tumour was completely excised with appropriate disease-free follow-up. Uncontrolled hypertension in the donor may have contributed to end-organ damage.

Q30. Option B – NG drainage, total parenteral nutrition and referral to a specialist unit

Prolonged peritoneal dialysis can lead to encapsulating peritoneal sclerosis (EPS). Fortunately, this is a rare complication, as it can be life-threatening. EPS manifests as severe fibrous changes of the peritoneum, leading to 'cocooning' of the bowel causing obstruction and eventually intestinal failure. Laparotomies in this patient population can be hazardous. Surgical treatment should be performed in specialised centres with an interest in EPS. EPS arises from long-standing inflammation and/or infection of the peritoneum in the context of PD.

Q31. Option E – ≥49

The UKELD score is derived from the patient's serum sodium, creatinine and bilirubin and the International Normalised Ratio (INR) of the prothrombin time. UKELD was developed in 2008 to risk-stratify liver transplant patients in the UK and predict waitlist mortality. UKELD≥49 is the minimum required score for chronic liver disease patients to be listed for liver transplantation. Estimated 1-year liver disease mortality without transplantation is >9% for a patient with a UKELD score of ≥49. A UKELD score of 60 indicates a 50% chance of 1-year survival.

This is not an absolute cut-off for all indications of a liver transplant. Special case scenarios such as HCC, and acute liver failure have separate individual protocols in place. Variant syndromes are presentations of CLD with UKELD<49. In case of variant syndromes or uncommon presentations, the transplant team can approach the National Appeals Panel for listing the patient for a liver transplant.

Q32. Option C – Serum Sodium

UKELD score is calculated from the patient's serum sodium, serum creatinine, serum bilirubin and INR.

Q33. Option E – All of the above

All of the above are indications for liver transplantation. As per the UK selection criteria, indications for a liver transplant can be broadly divided into chronic liver disease, acute liver failure, liver tumours and variant syndromes. Metabolic liver diseases with life-threatening extra-hepatic complications are an indication in children. Liver transplantation is usually offered if there is >50% probability of survival 5 years after transplantation with a quality of life acceptable to the patient and family.

Q34. Option A – Porto-pulmonary hypertension not responding to medical management

As per ODT liver transplant guidelines in the UK, there are two absolute contraindications to liver transplant: Non-adherence to alcohol abstinence and illicit drug use. Relative contraindications may preclude transplant in individual cases. While on the waitlist, primary disease progression or worsening of medical co-morbidities which is sufficient to impact the expected 50% survival at 5 years, mandates the de-selection of the patient from the waiting list. It could be temporary if there is room for optimisation of the condition, or permanent if the disease progression is irreversible.

In the above question, porto-pulmonary hypertension not responding to medical management is a contraindication to liver transplant as it is likely to reduce the survival of patients due to pulmonary hypertension. If diagnosed during the pre-transplant assessment, the patient should be referred to respiratory physicians. The rest of the options are variant syndromes where liver transplants can be indicated.

Q35. Option B – CT of the abdomen with contrast

In the immediate post-transplant period, worsening haemodynamic parameters with the need for increasing inotropic support, deteriorating LFTs and coagulation profile are indications that the transplanted liver is not functioning. Haemorrhagic drain output could be due to post-operative bleeding, however, it would not lead to significant deterioration in LFTs. In this scenario, high haemorrhagic drain output is an indication of worsening coagulopathy due to insufficient or absent synthetic function of the transplanted liver.

Causes of graft dysfunction in the immediate post-transplant period could be related to hepatic vascular inflow (hepatic artery thrombosis, portal venous thrombosis) or hepatic venous outflow obstruction. An immediate contrast CT scan should be done to exclude these vascular events. Graft dysfunction with good hepatic inflow/outflow is suggestive of primary non-function of the transplanted liver (diagnosis of exclusion). A patient diagnosed with PNF should be listed for re-transplant on an emergency basis. In the UK, these patients are listed as super-urgent and are prioritised for organ allocation.

Q36. Option E – All of the above

During organ retrieval, it is not uncommon to encounter a severely atherosclerotic/calcified infra-renal aorta. Less commonly, the infra-renal aorta could be aneurysmal. Attempting to cannulate the infra-renal aorta increases the chances of intimal dissection, which can extend into the arteries of organs to be transplanted, and/or poor perfusion of organs with a preservation fluid.

In either case, when faced with such a situation, cannulation can be done in either of the common iliac or external iliac arteries. A smaller size cannula may be needed for these vessels and ligation of the contralateral common iliac artery, is important to prevent the flow of preservation fluid towards the lower limb.

If for any reason none of these major vessels in the abdomen are accessible or usable, antegrade cannulation of the thoracic aorta can be done coupled with ligation of the infra-renal aorta or bilateral common iliac arteries. Cardio-thoracic retrieval teams, if present, can help with this cannulation.

Q37. Option A – ERCP and stenting

Biliary reconstruction during a liver transplant could be performed by duct-to-duct anastomosis or Roux-en-y hepatico-jejunostomy anastomosis. Duct-to-duct anastomosis is the preferred technique as it prevents the reflux of intestinal contents into the transplant liver biliary tree, avoids an additional bowel anastomosis and the biliary system is accessible post-transplant by endoscopic approach (ERCP).

In the above-mentioned scenario, the biliary system can be accessed through ERCP. Cholangiography provides information about the extent of stricture. Balloon dilation ± stent placement can be performed, supported with IV antibiotics for treatment of cholangitis.

A combination of ERCP + PTBD (Rendezvous technique) can be undertaken for the management of complex or difficult-to-reach strictures.

Biliary complications are common post-transplant and are known to affect graft survival. Commonly noted biliary complications include biliary leaks/fistula, biliary strictures and cholangiopathy.

Q38. Option B – PTBD and stenting

Roux-en-Y hepatico-jejunostomy for biliary reconstruction during liver transplant is usually performed when the distal CBD on the recipient side is diseased or unsuitable for anastomosis as in portal biliopathy/PSC, or when there is a significant size discrepancy between the two ducts which can increase the chances of leaks/strictures. Distal jejuno-jejunostomy anastomosis is usually done about 50–60 cm distal to the duodenal-jejunal junction.

The most appropriate access to the biliary system of a transplanted liver with Roux-en-y anastomosis in place would be percutaneous transhepatic biliary drainage (PTBD) ± stenting.

Q39. Option A – Calculous cholecystitis is a common cause of biliary sepsis after a liver transplant

The donor gall bladder is generally removed during deceased donor liver transplantation as this is denervated and prone to the development of stone disease.

Biliary strictures can be classified as anastomotic or non-anastomotic. Non-anastomotic biliary strictures are usually located high up in the hilum. It is important to differentiate non-anastomotic strictures from cholangiopathy. Non-anastomotic strictures are commonly seen with DCD livers due to the ischaemic insult to the biliary system during the warm ischaemia time of DCD organ retrieval. Multiple such biliary strictures in the hilum and within the liver are suggestive of ischaemic cholangiopathy. It is important to exclude the recurrence of the primary liver disease as the cause of cholangiopathy.

A DCD liver from a donor age < 50 years, <10% steatosis, functional warm ischaemia time < 10 minutes and cold ischaemia time < 6–8 hours is considered an ideal DCD liver.

FURTHER READING

British Transplantation Society guidelines: Transplantation from deceased donors after circulatory death (Revised in 2018). https://bts.org.uk/guidelines-standards/

http://odt.nhs.uk/pdf/pancreas_selection_policy.pdf

https://assets.publishing.service.gov.uk/government/uploads/system/uploads/attachment_data/file/876161/SaBTO-microbiological-safety-guidelines.pd

https://assets.publishing.service.gov.uk/government/uploads/system/uploads/attachment_data/file/948068/transplantation_of_organs_from_deceased_donors_with_cancer_or_a_history_of_cancer-revised_FINAL44266_JNcw_cw.pdf

https://bts.org.uk/wp-content/uploads/2017/04/02_BTS_Kidney_Pancreas_HIV.pdf

https://bts.org.uk/wp-content/uploads/2018/03/BTS_HepB_Guidelines_FINAL_09.03.18.pdf

https://bts.org.uk/wp-content/uploads/2018/07/FINAL_LDKT-guidelines_June-2018.pdf

https://www.odt.nhs.uk/living-donation/uk-living-kidney-sharing-scheme/

Liver Transplantation: selection criteria and registration policy (POL 195/6). https://www.odt.nhs.uk/transplantation/tools-policies-and-guidance/policies-and-guidance/

López-Andújar R, Moya A, Montalvá E, Berenguer M, De Juan M, San Juan F, Pareja E, Vila JJ, Orbis F, Prieto M, Mir J. Lessons learned from anatomic variants of the hepatic artery in 1,081 transplanted livers. *Liver Transpl.* 2007 Oct;13(10):1401–4. doi: 10.1002/lt.21254.

Mittal S, Gough SC. Pancreas transplantation: a treatment option for people with diabetes. *Diabet Med.* 2014 May;31(5):512–21. doi: 10.1111/dme.12373.

Mittal S, Johnson P, Friend P. Pancreas transplantation: solid organ and islet. *Cold Spring Harb Perspect Med.* 2014 Apr 1;4(4):a015610. doi: 10.1101/cshperspect.a015610.

Neuberger J, Gimson A, Davies M, et al. Selection of patients for liver transplantation and allocation of donated livers in the UK. *Gut.* 2008;57(2):252–57.

Watson CJ, Harper SJ. Anatomical variation and its management in transplantation. *Am J Transplant.* 2015 Jun;15(6):1459–71. doi: 10.1111/ajt.13310.

13 Trauma Surgery

Tanvir Hossain

Q1. A 35-year-old lady is transferred from a DGH to MTC following RTC where she was knocked off her horse. Her HR is 89, BP is 116/90 and RR is 21. Her Hb is 121, platelet count is 345 and INR is 1.0. Trauma CT reports a grade 3 splenic injury, no contrast extravasation but some fluid in the left upper quadrant around the spleen. Select the most appropriate option from below.
- A. Laparotomy and splenectomy
- B. Observation at the surgical ward
- C. Splenic artery and vein embolisation
- D. Laparotomy and packing
- E. Level 2 care

Q2. A 70 kg pedestrian has been brought into the emergency department by paramedics after being hit by a motorcycle. Initial observations show a heart rate of 129, a BP of 90/70 and a RR of 30. She has a GCS of 15, and ABG shows a BE of −8. Which is the most likely estimated blood loss?
- A. 900 mL
- B. 1,150 mL
- C. 1,850 mL
- D. 2,670 mL
- E. 220 mL

Q3. A 63-year-old man is brought into the emergency department after RTC with a RR of 34, a HR of 119, a BP of 92/60 and reduced air entry in the left chest, distended neck veins, and 02 saturation of 89%. What is the next management?
- A. Chest drain in the left fifth intercostal space mid-axillary line
- B. Needle pericardiocentesis
- C. Needle decompression into the left second intercostal space
- D. Needle decompression in the left fifth intercostal space mid-axillary line
- E. IV fluid resuscitation

Q4. Which of the following is not an indication of an emergency thoracotomy?
- A. Over 1,500 mL immediate blood loss following chest drain insertion
- B. Traumatic thoracic injury with unresponsive hypotension
- C. Patients with ongoing bleeding from a chest drain of 200 mL/h for 2–4 hours
- D. No ROSC after 1 minute of CPR following witnessing a blunt traumatic injury
- E. Witnessed cardiac arrest following traumatic thoracic injury and after 2 minutes of closed CPR including bilateral chest decompression

DOI: 10.1201/9781003221234-13

Q5. A 31-year-old man was involved in a RTC whilst riding his e-scooter. Three days following laparotomy for a small bowel injury and also external fixation of a left tibia/fibula fracture, he became tachypnoeic, hypoxic and oliguric. His heart rate is 110, BP is 110/80, O_2 saturation is 88 and ABG shows a PaO_2 of 6.9 kPa.
Select the most likely diagnosis.
A. Further intra-abdominal bleeding
B. Chest consolidation
C. Fat embolism
D. Pulmonary Embolism
E. Head injury not previously noted

Q6. A 49-year-old man with a BMI of 42 has had an RTC whereby a lorry struck his motorcycle. Paramedics intubated him at the roadside. He is brought into the emergency department, and at the primary survey, his heart rate is 45 with a BP of 201/119. His neck is fully immobilised, and the collar has not allowed you to assess neck veins. What is the most likely diagnosis?
A. Spinal cord injury
B. Cardiac tamponade
C. Tension pneumothorax
D. Use of beta-blockers
E. Head injury

Q7. A 43-year-old cyclist has collided with an e-scooter and sustained an obvious head injury and trauma. The CT scan shows a grade 4 spleen injury and liver laceration; his HR is 140, BP is 83/52 and RR is 28. What is your management strategy?
A. Resuscitate with blood products and, if responding, refer to neurosurgery
B. Trauma laparotomy
C. Refer to interventional radiology for embolisation of the splenic artery
D. Fluid resuscitation with crystalloids and, if responding, refer to neurosurgery
E. Refer to interventional radiology for embolisation of bleeding point at liver and splenic artery

Q8. A 53-year-old man is in a RTC and is taken for a trauma laparotomy due to hypotension and peritonism. At laparotomy a bucket handle small bowel tear is repaired, and you find a deep liver laceration to the right lobe of the liver actively bleeding. How would you proceed?
A. Call the HPB team and arrange the right hemihepatectomy
B. Close the abdomen and arrange angioembolisation in the radiology department
C. Ensure the patient is on a carbon fibre-top operating table and call interventional radiology for help
D. Trial of a maximum of two different haemostatic agents of increasing volume into the tear until bleeding stops
E. Pack the liver into anatomical shape and employ a temporary dressing on the abdomen and organise a re-look laparotomy in 48 hours with close observation

Q9. A 41-year-old cyclist swerves to avoid a cat and collides with the kerb and is catapulted into the handlebars and then onto the concrete pavement hitting his head. A Bastion protocol CT scan finds a splenic laceration involving the hilum, with a contrast blush. The patient is haemodynamically stable but complains of left upper quadrant pain. What is your next step?

A. Observe in level 2 care
B. Observe in level 2 care and repeat CT angiogram within 24 hours
C. Laparotomy and splenectomy
D. Splenic artery embolisation
E. Admit to level 1 care and observe with serial Hb check, examination and vital signs, with imaging if any concerns with the above

Q10. A 19-year-old lady is ejected from her bicycle and lands on a bollard. She initially goes home but due to increased pain attends the emergency department where she is tachycardic. A Bastion protocol CT scan shows peripancreatic fluids and disruption at the head of the pancreas; there is also some free fluid in the abdomen and at laparotomy, there is a small perforation at the proximal jejunum where the tissue is healthy and viable. What is your management choice?

A. Repair small bowel and resect pancreatic injury
B. Resect perforated bowel but do not anastomose and organise a re-look in 48 hours
C. Washout, resection of the small bowel and distal pancreatectomy and splenectomy
D. Washout, drains placed around the head of the pancreas and primary closure of small bowel injury
E. Washout, primary closure of small bowel injury as a definitive procedure

Q11. A 37-year-old man is involved in an altercation and pushed in front of a moving white van. He has multiple injuries including fractures right humerus, a large bruise across his abdomen and tachycardia of 112. On arrival at the emergency department, he has bp 118/67 HR 110 following a unit of blood administered by the paramedic team. Arterial blood gas shows a Hb of 72. What is your next step?

A. Reduce his fracture
B. Secure airway
C. Place blocks to reinforce the c-spine immobilisation
D. Request urgent Trauma CT scan
E. Activate major haemorrhage protocol

Q12. A 21-year-old male intoxicated driver is involved in a collision with a large tree. He is restrained with airbags activated and is brought to the emergency department physiologically stable. Trauma laparotomy is done for contrast extravasation from small bowel mesentery on a CT scan. A small bowel mesenteric tear is primarily suture repaired. Day 2 post op he is complaining of increasing pain and a CT scan shows mesenteric haematoma. Continued pain leads to a repeat CT 24 hours later showing this haematoma to be increased. He also has dilated small bowel throughout. Describe the best management option.

A. Return to theatre for relaparotomy
B. NG tube for ileus
C. Liaise with interventional radiology for embolisation
D. Observe as the phenomena is self-limiting
E. Laparoscopy and endoclip to just below the haematoma

Q13. A 23-year-old man has been assaulted after an altercation at a football match. He has severe left-sided chest and upper abdominal pain. He is physiologically stable and pain has improved with opiate analgesia. A trauma CT scan performed at 11.30 pm that night found three nondisplaced rib fractures of the left 7th, 8th and 9th ribs. No pneumothorax. He is needing 2 L of O_2 via nasal cannula to maintain satisfactory oxygen saturations. How would you manage this patient?

A. Discharge with an oxycodone prescription
B. Organise epidural
C. Refer to orthopaedics for rib fixation
D. Admit and observe
E. Admit and liaise with the pain management team for infusion with PCA

Q14. An 18-year-old female is stabbed with a letter opener in the left chest just below the level of the nipple. She has a GCS of 15/15, heart rate of 100 and bp of 108/65. O_2 sat. is 92% and RR is 25. She is hyperresonant to chest percussion with a dull left base and a chest tube was placed for presumed haemopneumothorax. She was commenced on a bag of crystalloids. What is the next step in management?

A. Insert right-sided ICD
B. CT chest abdomen pelvis
C. Re-examine the chest
D. FAST scan
E. Thoracotomy if the blood output is >1,500 mL

Q15. A 23-year-old man is stabbed in the right chest with a small knife. He is tachypneic with a RR of 25. His HR is 126, and his BP is 82/53. His neck veins do not appear distended. There is good air entry bilaterally on chest auscultation but dull to percussion at the bases. What is the likely diagnosis?

A. Haemothorax
B. Pericardial tamponade
C. Pneumothorax
D. Lung injury
E. Shock from liver injury

Q16. A 38-year-old lady with a BMI of 42 is unstrained and involved in an RTA. Her GCS is 8. Prior to transfer to a CT scanner, what is essential?

A. Appropriate sedative drugs
B. Definitive airway
C. Fast Scan
D. NG tube
E. CXR

Q17. A 43-year-old motorcyclist is admitted following a collision with deer. He has severe abdominal pain but is physiologically normal, and his abdomen is soft on examination. What is the most specific test to assess solid organ injury in the abdomen?

A. Clinical examination
B. US Abdo
C. MRI
D. Diagnostic peritoneal lavage
E. CT of the abdomen/pelvis

Q18. A 30-year-old lady who is 32 weeks pregnant has a fallen down half a flight of stairs. She has a GCS of 15/15 and has normal observations. She has mild generalised abdominal pain and distention. Which one of the following statements is true regarding a pregnant patient who presents following blunt trauma?
  A. Clinical signs of peritoneal irritation are less evident in pregnant women
  B. Blood loss of 1.5 L will certainly exhibit signs and symptoms of hypovolemia in late pregnancy
  C. Early gastric decompression is contraindicated
  D. The majority of injury in pregnancy is penetrating injury
  E. A lap belt alone is the best form of restraint due to the size of the gravid uterus

Q19. Class II shock is characterised by:
  A. Reduced blood pressure
  B. Increased pulse pressure
  C. Mildly increased respiratory rate
  D. No need for blood products
  E. Base deficit of up to -6 HCO_3^-

Q20. A 56-year-old lorry driver fell asleep at the wheel at 70 mph. The automatic braking system failed to stop a collision but reduced the speed such that the impact was at 30 mph. On arrival, he was alert with GCS 15/15 and tachycardic at 110 with normal blood pressure. He complains of left upper quadrant pain and was found to have pneumoperitoneum after the Bastion protocol CT trauma series. What is your diagnosis?
  A. Grade 1–4 splenic rupture
  B. Liver laceration
  C. DJ flexure rupture
  D. IVC injury
  E. Diaphragmatic injury

Q21. A 28-year-old otherwise fit and well cyclist collides with a pedestrian and lands on a parking restriction bollard. He is unstable in the emergency department and was taken directly for a trauma laparotomy. He is found to have multiple small bowel mesentery tears, a transected left colon and a pelvic haematoma thought to be from a pelvic fracture. What is your course of action?
  A. Damage control surgery
  B. Suture bleeding points, and if all bowel appears healthy, primary anastomosis and closure of the abdomen
  C. Pack pelvis, colostomy
  D. Resect devascularised small bowel with primary anastomosis, colostomy, fixation of pelvic fractures
  E. Primary bowel anastomosis and call interventional radiology

Q22. A 37-year-old lady falls off her 15-hand horse which subsequently lands on her. She is brought to the emergency department in a scoop with c-spine immobilised and haemodynamically stable but peritonitic. Upon laparotomy, she is found to have two small bowel injuries, bruising to the small bowel mesentery and a diaphragmatic rupture in the left upper quadrant. The small bowel injuries were amenable to primary repair. How do you manage the diaphragmatic injury?

A. The damage has been controlled, return to intensive care ASAP and organise repair in 48 hours

B. Primary closure

C. Close the abdomen and repair the diaphragm when a biological mesh is available

D. Buttress the repair for prolene mesh

E. No action, organise repair of diaphragm electively with a specialist surgeon

Q23. A 43-year-old man is involved in an altercation in a pub car park. His shirt is bloodied, and paramedics find that he has been stabbed in the lower abdomen. The major trauma team arranges an emergency laparotomy where he is found to have a 1.5 cm colonic injury on the anterior side of the caecum with a small amount of surrounding contamination. How do you manage this?

A. Limited right hemicolectomy

B. Primary repair and defunctioning loop ileostomy

C. Primary repair only

D. T-tube

E. Exteriorise the defect as a stoma

Q24. A 17-year-old cyclist is undergoing laparotomy and splenectomy following a collision rupturing her spleen. The major trauma fellow is struggling with haemostasis and is unsure if she has control of the splenic vein. What are the key anatomic relations to help her?

A. Splenic vein is anterior to and along the superior border of the pancreas

B. Splenic vein lies anterior to the tail of the pancreas

C. Inferior mesenteric vein will drain into the splenic vein

D. Splenic vein joins SMV to form the hepatic portal vein

E. Splenic vein is posterior to the tail of the pancreas

Q25. A 38-year-old lady of BMI 35 is stabbed by her partner multiple times with injuries to her left forearm, and shoulder and a stab wound into her right upper quadrant. A contrast-enhanced CT scan shows a small amount of free air near the peritoneum at the site of entry but no obvious peritoneal breach. The patient is tender at the site of the wound but not peritonitic and physiologically stable. How do you manage this case?

A. Serial abdominal examinations

B. Repeat CT scan within 24 hours

C. Diagnostic laparoscopy

D. Trauma laparotomy

E. Diagnostic laparoscopy in 24 hours

ANSWERS

Q1. Option E – Level 2 care.

A haemodynamically stable patient with grade 3 splenic injury can be managed non-operatively; however, she requires careful close observation and hence level 2 care. Grade 3 splenic injury in haemodynamically stable patients can also undergo splenic artery embolisation, and this intervention is increasingly becoming favoured, especially in patients too frail for surgery.

Q2. Option C – 1,850 mL.

The patient's parameters match with ATLS tenth edition shock classification class 3.

Q3. Option D – Needle decompression in the left fifth intercostal space mid-axillary line.

ATLS tenth edition now recommends this for decompression of tension pneumothorax due to studies showing improved success in entering the thoracic cavity from here. If a needle compression fails here due to the haemothorax or the catheter being kinked, a finger thoracostomy is advised. Chest drains of 28–32F are advised for drainage.

Q4. Option D – No ROSC after 1 minute of CPR following witnessed blunt traumatic injury.

The tenth edition ATLS course advocates thoracotomy and vertical pericardiotomy if there is no ROSC after closed CPR and bilateral chest decompression for up to 3 minutes.

Q5. Option C – Fat embolism.

Fat embolisms usually present 2–3 days following injury or surgery, in contrast to pulmonary embolisms which are typically 7 days following an event. The presentation may be dyspnoea, oliguria and confusion. There may be a petechial rash over the neck and axillae. Fat globules may be seen in the retina and noted in sputum and urine.

Q6. Option E – Head injury.

Head injury. Cushing's triad: Hypertension (with widened pulse pressure), bradycardia and irregular respirations.

Q7. Option B – Trauma laparotomy.

An unstable patient with grade 4 splenic injury is likely actively bleeding and needs urgent laparotomy

Q8. Option E – Pack the liver into anatomical shape and employ a temporary dressing on the abdomen and organise a re-look laparotomy in 48 hours with close observation.

Q9. Option D – Splenic artery embolisation.

Laparotomy and splenectomy would be considered if the patient was haemodynamically unstable, unresponsive to resuscitation or peritonic. Splenic artery embolisation where this is a contrast blush or injury to the hilum can lower the chance of the case progressing to needing surgery.

Q10. Option D – Washout, drains placed around the head of the pancreas and primary closure of small bowel injury.

Distal pancreatic injuries can be resected but the head of pancreas injuries are preferred to have drains placed, although there is the potential in re-look surgery to have completion of Whipple's procedure but rarely in the initial damage control phase. Small bowel injuries that are small and tissue is viable with patent blood supply can be primarily closed.

Q11. Option D – Request urgent trauma CT scan.

He is haemodynamically stable with a unit of blood; it would be prudent to get a CT scan to identify his injuries to plan further management

Q12. Option A – Return to theatre for re-laparotomy.

The repeat CT shows worsening signs and a re-look laparotomy is warranted, and there may be a risk to small bowel viability if any continued bleeding is not controlled.

Q13. Option B – Organise epidural.

Rib fractures of four or more usually warrant epidural analgesia. Although this young otherwise fit patient has only three rib fractures that are undisplaced, and his pain is apparently well controlled with opiates, he still has an oxygen requirement; therefore, a step up to epidural may help.

Q14. Option C – Re-examine the chest.

Interventions should be followed by re-examination to confirm improvement and consider any other new findings.

Q15. Option E – Shock from liver injury.

Lack of neck vein distention and good air entry, along with shock make heavy bleeding from a liver injury more probable.

Q16. Option B – Definitive airway.

The patient needs to be safe for transfer to the CT scanner. It is best practice to use a checklist to confirm the safe transfer and GCS 8 would warrant a definitive airway.

Q17. Option E – CT of the abdomen/pelvis.

CT is the gold standard in this scenario, especially in a patient stable enough for transfer to a CT scanner.

Q18. Option A – Clinical signs of peritoneal irritation are less evident in pregnant women.

Blood loss of 1.2–1.5 L may not necessarily exhibit signs as blood volume increases throughout pregnancy. Early gastric decompression is advised to prevent aspiration in light of delayed gastric emptying. Blunt injury makes up over 90% of abdominal injuries in the pregnant population. A lap belt may cause uterine rupture especially if worn high over the uterus and in particular if not in conjunction with a shoulder belt to share the force and prevent flexing over the uterus.

Q19. Option E – A base deficit of up to −6 HCO_3^-.

Class II shock whereby 15%–30% of blood volume is lost may exhibit tachycardia but blood pressure, urine output, respiratory rate and GCS may remain stable. A base deficit may be between −2 to −6. The ATLS tenth edition shock classification states that class II shock may exhibit a reduced pulse pressure.

Q20. Option C – DJ flexure rupture.

The free air raises suspicion of visceral injury

Q21. Option A – Damage control surgery.

With multiple injuries and a question of small bowel viability after achieving haemostasis, damage control surgery is the safest option, this could mean avoiding small bowel resection and if the patient is stable anastomosis for the transected colon.

Q22. Option B – Primary closure.

Diaphragmatic injuries can be primarily repaired unless the patient is unstable or other injuries are extensive enough to warrant a damage control approach. A mesh is not usually necessary for these injuries.

Q23. Option C – Primary repair only.

A small clean injury with no signs of ischaemia can be primarily repaired if the defect goes beyond 50% of the circumference of the colon resection is mandated. These injuries should always be inspected to identify an exit point of the knife. If the injury was more distal in the colon, the merits and risks of primary closure in an unprepared colon must be considered.

Q24. Option E – Splenic vein is posterior to the tail of the pancreas.

The most relevant landmark in this scenario is nearest to the spleen, where pancreatic injuries also take place and care must be taken during dissection, particularly when getting control of bleeding. The splenic artery runs anterior to and along the superior border of the pancreas.

Q25. Option C – Diagnostic laparoscopy.

Physiological changes may be exhibited only when there is significant peritonitis or bleeding. A CT scan in 24 hours may show free fluid or more free air if there is bowel injury; however, there is no guarantee. A laparoscopy would be able to exclude a genuine peritoneal breach; if no such breach has occurred, then no further action is required; however, if there is a breach, then depending on one's skill set, one can proceed to complete evaluation of the abdomen either laparoscopically or through conversion to laparotomy.

14 Vascular Surgery

Mohamed Baguneid, Hussien Rabee, and Sulaiman Saif Salim Alshamsi

Q1. A 28-year-old woman presents with large varicose veins in her left leg. She experiences aching in her left leg that is worse at the end of the day and is associated with itching. She had a previous left femoral fracture 5 years ago which was treated with a femoral intra-medullary nail. Which of the following statements would be correct?

A. Advise her to wear Class 2 above-knee compression stockings and elevate her leg when possible

B. Recommend a left sapheno-femoral junction ligation, stripping of the great saphenous vein and multiple phlebectomy

C. Arrange a venous duplex scan of her left leg, and if there is evidence of great saphenous vein reflux, recommend endovenous ablation therapy

D. Perform a hand-held Doppler test in the clinic, and if there is reflux in the sapheno-femoral junction, then recommend endovenous ablation therapy

E. Reassure the patient that she does not need treatment at the present time and advise that she should exercise more and take 75 mg of aspirin daily

Q2. A 75-year-old man presented to the emergency department with a 6-hour history of a cold, painful and pulseless right leg. He had severe chest and back pains the day before. On admission, his blood pressure was 210/110 mmHg and his pulse rate was 88 bpm with a sinus rhythm. A chest X-ray shows a widened mediastinum and ECG was unremarkable. What is the best initial course of action?

A. Give 5,000 u of unfractionated heparin bolus, and take the patient as an emergency to theatre for a right femoral embolectomy

B. Give opiate analgesia and start a GTN infusion. Arrange an urgent arterial duplex scan of his right leg

C. Give opiate analgesia and arrange for a labetalol infusion with a target systolic pressure of 100 mmHg and pulse rate of 60 bpm

D. Arrange immediate CT angiogram of the aorta and lower-limb arteries and transfer the patient to intensive care or coronary care unit

E. Take the patient immediately to the vascular interventional suite for aortography and emergency placement of a thoracic endovascular stent graft

Q3. A 70-year-old man presents with claudication in both gluteal, thigh and calf muscles at around 200 m. It has been present for 5 years but worsened slightly in the past 6 months. He still manages to walk to his local shopping centre but feels he has to stop frequently *en route*. He is a lifelong smoker and has type 2 diabetes with an HbA1c of 7.8%. Which of the following statements is most accurate?

DOI: 10.1201/9781003221234-14

A. He has atherosclerotic disease affecting his aorto-iliac arteries and should have a CT angiogram of his aorta and lower-limb arteries to evaluate his occlusive disease further prior to offering surgical or endovascular reconstruction.

B. He should start on an antiplatelet agent and a statin and be advised to stop smoking. He should have a review of his diabetes management and see a podiatrist for foot care. No imaging is necessary, and he is advised to attend a supervised exercise programme.

C. He has an aorto-iliac occlusive disease and should have an arterial duplex scan and be referred for aorto-iliac artery stenting after starting antiplatelet and statin therapy.

D. Refer to a cardiologist for secondary cardiovascular prevention therapy and perform ankle brachial pressure index (ABPI) measurements. If ABPI <0.5, he must have a CT angiogram of his aorta and lower-limb arteries prior to revascularisation.

E. He should be started on dual antiplatelet therapy and a statin. An arterial duplex scan of both lower limbs is required to plan for possible endovascular treatment.

Q4. A 78-year-old woman presents with a 4-hour history of a cold painful left hand. She lives on her own at home and is independent and active. She was found to be in atrial fibrillation on arrival and with no brachial, radial or ulnar pulse on the left. She had normal pulses in her right hand and both feet. What would be the best initial management?

A. Give 5,000 u bolus of unfractionated heparin, arrange an immediate arterial duplex scan and take her to the theatre to perform a brachial embolectomy under local anaesthesia

B. Start a heparin and prostacyclin infusion and provide analgesia. Convert to warfarin when pain in left arm improves

C. Urgent review by a cardiologist for cardioversion to correct atrial fibrillation prior to performing a brachial embolectomy

D. Arrange a CT angiogram of the arch of the aorta and left upper limb and proceed with catheter-directed thrombolysis

E. Take the patient to the theatre for urgent left brachial embolectomy and forearm fasciotomy. Transfer patient to high dependency unit and start a heparin infusion post-op.

Q5. A 58-year-old woman attends your clinic for follow-up having had an abdominal ultrasound scan for presumed gallstone disease. Her liver function tests were normal, but the ultrasound report noted several small gallstones in a thin-walled gallbladder with no biliary dilatation. You note a comment in the report of a 4.9 cm infra-renal abdominal aortic aneurysm (AAA). During the clinic visit, she mentions that she has also been suffering from back pain for the last 3 weeks. On examining her abdomen, you note that she had very mild discomfort on deep palpation in the epigastric region, but her abdomen was otherwise soft and she had palpable peripheral pulses. What is your best course of action:

A. Arrange for a laparoscopic cholecystectomy on your elective list and refer to the vascular surgeons to arrange surveillance of her AAA

B. Refer to vascular surgeons to be seen in their next available clinic prior to listing for a laparoscopic cholecystectomy

    C.   Arrange an urgent outpatient CT scan of the AAA and refer to vascular surgeons

    D.   Recommend that she is admitted from the clinic under vascular surgeons with the view to the treatment of her 4.9 cm infra-renal AAA

    E.   Reassure the patient that her gallstones do not require treatment and arrange a repeat ultrasound of her AAA in 3 months, and if they are >5.5 cm in diameter, refer to vascular surgeons for treatment

Q6. A 63-year-old man with well-controlled type 2 diabetes and hypertension suffered transient weakness in his right arm and leg 3 days earlier which has now fully recovered. He had a carotid duplex scan at a private health screening centre which demonstrated 90% right internal carotid artery stenosis and 65% left internal carotid artery stenosis. Both vertebral arteries demonstrated normal orthograde blood flow. Which of the following management options is most accurate?

    A.   Start the patient on an antiplatelet agent and statin. Repeat carotid duplex scan at a specialised vascular centre, and if findings are similar arrange for urgent left carotid endarterectomy within 2 weeks of his initial symptoms

    B.   Start the patient on an antiplatelet agent and statin. Arrange a CT angiogram of his carotid at a specialised vascular centre and if the right carotid artery is still 90% stenosed, arrange for urgent right carotid endarterectomy within 2 weeks of his initial symptoms

    C.   Start the patient on dual antiplatelets and a statin. Repeat the carotid duplex scan and arrange a CT angiogram of his carotid artery and plan for an urgent left carotid stent

    D.   Start patient on heparin infusion, repeat carotid duplex scan at a specialised vascular centre with the view to performing an urgent left carotid endarterectomy

    E.   Start patient on a heparin infusion and admit for an urgent carotid angiogram with a view to bilateral carotid stents

Q7. A 60-year-old man presents with a 6-month history of postprandial abdominal pain and unintentional weight loss of 10 kg. He is a lifelong smoker and has a chronic renal disease (CKD stage 4). He has been extensively investigated by gastroenterologists with upper and lower GI endoscopies that were normal. A CT scan (without contrast) was ordered and showed a severe calcified aorta and origins of the coeliac and superior mesenteric artery origins, but no other abnormalities were seen. What would be a reasonable approach to his management?

    A.   Arrange further blood tests for tumour markers and a PET scan

    B.   Arrange for a CT with contrast in the mesenteric phase

    C.   Arrange a diagnostic catheter angiogram to assess the coeliac, superior and inferior mesenteric arteries as well as internal iliac arteries

    D.   Arrange an arterial duplex of the coeliac, superior and inferior mesenteric arteries to assess for any significant stenoses

    E.   Arrange for a laparotomy with the view to evaluating the bowel and performing superior mesenteric artery bypass

Q8. A 34-year-old semi-professional female swimmer presented with a 2-day history of acute left upper limb swelling. She is otherwise well with no previous history of deep vein thrombosis and no family history of thrombosis. There is no recent history of trauma or upper limb venous cannulation. Which of the following statements is correct:
   A. She needs to be admitted for an urgent venogram and antiplatelet therapy
   B. An MRI scan should be performed to assess her thoracic outlet prior to starting anticoagulation
   C. She should start anticoagulation immediately, and an arterial duplex scan must be performed to rule out a subclavian artery aneurysm
   D. Anticoagulation should be commenced immediately and a venous duplex scan must be performed to establish if she has an axillary and subclavian vein thrombosis
   E. She should undergo urgent thoracic outlet decompression with thrombectomy of likely axillary vein thrombosis.

Q9. A 45-year-old man presented to the clinic having had an ultrasound scan in a private health care facility, demonstrating an AAA measuring 6.8 cm in maximal diameter. He has no significant past medical history apart from well-controlled hypertension. He has two brothers who have had surgery for full AAAs in the past. Which of the following statement is correct:
   A. The patient should have a computerised tomography scan with arterial phase contrast and undergo cardiovascular risk assessment prior to being offered open surgery for his large AAA.
   B. The patient should have an echocardiogram and chest X-ray as the prominence of his preoperative assessment prior to undergoing endovascular repair of his AAA.
   C. The patient should undergo endovascular stent graft repair of his AAA as it carries a low perioperative mortality rate and provides a durable repair for a long time.
   D. The patient should have a repeat ultrasound of his AAA in a specialist vascular stent. If his ultrasound is consistent with the scan he had in a private healthcare facility, then he should be off it in urgent open surgical repair of his AAA within 2 weeks.
   E. The family history of AAAs suggests that he may have a collagen vascular disorder which will require further investigation before considering surgical repair.

Q10. A 35-year-old female patient presents to the clinic with tender inflamed varicose veins in her right leg. The pain in her right leg started 1 week ago and extends from her knee to the mid-thigh on its medial aspect. She has no other medical problems and does not take the oral contraceptive pill. She has had varicose veins for many years which have not caused any problems. Which of the following statements would be considered a suitable management plan:
   A. She should undergo surgical treatment of her varicose veins that would include disconnection of her right sapheno-femoral junction stripping of the great saphenous vein and multiple phlebectomy.
   B. She should be commenced on oral anticoagulation and given class 2 above-knee graduated compression stockings.

C.   Should be advised to elevate the leg and take nonsteroidal anti-inflammatory medications (NSAIDs).

D.   A venous duplex scan should be performed to establish the extent of superficial thrombophlebitis and she should be recommended to wear class 2 graduated above-knee compression stockings and take nonsteroidal anti-inflammatory drugs (NSAIDs). Once superficial thrombophlebitis has settled down, she should be considered for treatment of her superficial venous insufficiency.

E.   She should be admitted for bed rest and leg elevation and a venogram performed to confirm whether she has suffered a deep vein thrombosis.

Q11. A 74-year-old lady with a 6-year history of a nonhealing right ankle venous ulcer presents to the clinic. The ulcer is not painful but has become slightly larger in size over the past 2 months despite treatment with leg-graduated compression bandaging. Which of the following would be considered appropriate management:

A.   Patient should be advised to continue with four-layer graduated compression bandaging for a further 8 weeks and also commenced on a 2-week course of antibiotics.

B.   Patient should have an arterial duplex scan and a CT angiogram to check for any signs of arterial disease before re-applying compression bandaging.

C.   The patient should undergo superficial venous surgery to speed up the healing of her venous leg ulcer.

D.   The patient should be commenced on a 2-week course of antibiotics and advised to elevate their leg.

E.   Patient should be reassessed with the ABPI being measured and a biopsy of the edge of the ulcer being performed. A venous duplex scan would be recommended prior to considering any form of superficial venous treatment.

Q12. A 64-year-old man developed a swelling in the right groin following cardiac catheterisation through the right femoral artery the previous day. The patient had a coronary stent and was commenced on dual antiplatelet therapy for a non-ST-elevation myocardial infarction. The cardiologist performed an ultrasound scan, confirming a 3.5 cm pseudoaneurysm of the femoral artery. What is the best option for his management:

A.   Repeat the arterial duplex scan in 1 week to see if it has thrombosed by itself post-op.

B.   Stop the patient's antiplatelet therapy and compress the groin swelling for 24 hours prior to repeating the ultrasound scan.

C.   Patient should go to surgery on an urgent basis for full ligation of the femoral artery aneurysm with a short interposition bypass graft.

D.   The patient should undergo an endovascular procedure to insist on a covered stent graft into the common femoral artery to seal the false aneurysm from the inside.

E.   Ultrasound-guided compression of the false aneurysm for at least 20 minutes should be attempted, and if this fails to thrombose the false aneurysm, then ultrasound-guided thrombin injection should be performed.

Q13. A 74-year-old gentleman with COPD presents with a 3-day history of critical lower-limb ischaemia in his left lower limb following a 2-year history of claudication. A CT angiogram revealed a 4.8 cm AAA with a large amount of mural thrombus and a complete occlusion of the left common and external iliac arteries. His right iliac system was widely patent with normal femoral, popliteal and calf arteries. The best management option is:

A. Left iliac thrombectomy and bifurcated standard EVAR.
B. Left iliac thrombectomy and duplex scan follow-up for AAA.
C. Right-to-left fem-fem crossover bypass and duplex scan follow-up for AAA.
D. Aorto-uni-iliac EVAR and right-to left femoro-femoral crossover bypass.
E. Aorto-uni-iliac EVAR.

Q14. A 64-year-old gentleman presented with a 12-month history of a 3×7 cm superficial ulcer at the left leg gaiter area with palpable pulses. PMH: bilateral DVT, HTN and IHD. The best management is:

A. Compression bandage dressing and follow-up for ulcer healing.
B. Venous duplex scan, compression bandage dressing and endovenous ablation for superficial varicosities only if deep veins are patent.
C. Venous duplex scan, Compression bandage dressing and endovenous ablation for superficial varicosities only if deep veins are competent.
D. Compression bandage dressing and venous Duplex scan after complete ulcer healing.
E. Venous duplex scan, endovenous ablation for superficial varicosities only if deep veins are patent, leg elevation and non-compressible daily dressing.

Q15. A 54-year-old lady presented with acute left upper limb swelling due to subclavian DVT. The swelling responded reasonably with anticoagulation. Scanning proved to have a cervical rib causing venous compression and thoracic outlet syndrome (TOS). How would you manage further?

A. Oral anticoagulation for 6 months and conservative management for TOS because the complication has already happened.
B. No need for anticoagulation as upper limb DVT is unlikely to cause PE.
C. Oral anticoagulation for 6 months and decompression of the TOS only if duplex scan demonstrated venous recanalisation.
D. Oral anticoagulation for 6 months and urgent decompression of the TOS.
E. Urgent subclavian vein stenting, Oral anticoagulation for 6 months and decompression of the TOS at the end of anticoagulation.

Q16. A 47-year-old gentleman was admitted to the ICU following a traumatic car accident and ventilated for head trauma. The right leg showed multiple bruises, but no fractures were detected. The limb is swollen, tender and well-perfused and normal pedal pulses were palpable. On the second day, the limb was the same but more tender and painful. The most appropriate line of management is:

A. Consider fasciotomy as soon as possible.
B. Consider fasciotomy if the compartment pressure is 35 mmHg or higher.
C. Consider fasciotomy if the compartment pressure is 20 mmHg or higher.
D. Consider fasciotomy if CT angiogram reveals compartment syndrome.
E. Consider fasciotomy if pedal pulses disappear.

Q17. A 68-year-old right-handed lady presented with dysphasia and right leg weakness for 45 minutes. CT scan did not show cerebral infarction. She was seen by the TIA clinic 7 weeks later due to COVID-19 scan restrictions which recommended a change of her daily aspirin to clopidogrel and adding statins with better control of blood pressure. Then, a carotid duplex scan confirmed 60%–69%. What is the most appropriate management?

A. Left carotid endarterectomy CEA if CT angiogram confirms significant stenosis.

B. Left carotid endarterectomy CEA as a duplex scan based on velocity is more accurate.

C. Left carotid endarterectomy CEA is less complicated with aspirin and not clopidogrel.

D. Left carotid endarterectomy CEA is less beneficial after 6 weeks post-event and the best medical therapy is enough to manage this lady.

E. Left carotid endarterectomy CEA is only indicated with residual neurological deficit.

Q18. A 79-year-old gentleman presented to the A&E department with abdominal pain, signs of shock, and pulsatile abdominal swelling. The next step is:

A. Ultrasound scan to confirm ruptured AAA

B. Ultrasound scan to confirm AAA

C. CT scan to confirm AAA

D. CT scan to confirm ruptured AAA

E. Urgent laparotomy if the patient is known to have 5.5 cm AAA or higher

Q19. All the following are indications of IVC filter EXCEPT:

A. Unilateral extensive iliofemoral DVT.

B. Bilateral DVT with recent peptic ulcer bleeding.

C. Unilateral DVT with recent head trauma.

D. Bilateral DVT with failure of anticoagulation.

E. Unilateral DVT with heparin-induced thrombocytopenia.

Q20. A 62-year-old lady with PMH of ex-smoking and HTN presented with deteriorating right lower-limb claudication over the last 3 years. Currently, she has left foot rest pain with a tiny ulcer. CT angiogram confirmed total occlusion for the left common iliac artery and multi-level severe stenosis of the left external iliac artery. All other vessels are reasonably patent. The best line of treatment is:

A. Right-to-left fem-fem crossover bypass.

B. Left axillo-femoral bypass.

C. Left iliac arteries remote endarterectomy.

D. Left aorto-femoral bypass.

E. Thrombolysis with angioplasty of residual stenosis.

ANSWERS

Q1. Option C – Arrange a venous duplex scan of her left leg and if there is evidence of great saphenous vein reflux, recommend endovenous ablation therapy.

This patient is suffering from symptoms typical of venous hypertension associated with varicose veins. However, her history of a previous femoral fracture raises the suspicion of old deep vein thrombosis and possible deep venous insufficiency. A venous duplex scan is obligatory if varicose vein treatment is to be considered. It helps establish the anatomy of her venous system as well as confirm deep venous patency and whether there is reflux in either the superficial or deep venous systems. If she has superficial venous reflux, she would be best treated by endovenous ablation therapy (e.g., laser or radiofrequency ablation). If she is not suitable for endovenous ablation therapy, then foam sclerotherapy can be considered or traditional surgical procedures like sapheno-femoral junction ligation and long saphenous vein stripping. This is in accordance with NICE clinical guidelines CG168, 2013.

Q2. Option C – Give opiate analgesia and arrange for a labetalol infusion with a target systolic pressure of 100 mmHg and a pulse rate of 60 bpm.

The patient clearly presents with acute limb ischaemia. The fact that the question states a 6-hour history raises the question that there is very little time left before his leg becomes irreversibly ischaemic. There are many causes for acute limb ischaemia including embolus, trauma and thrombosis of popliteal artery aneurysms. However, this patient presented with chest pain, hypertension and a widened mediastinum which raises the suspicion of aortic dissection. Aortic dissections can cause acute limb ischaemia. Whilst it is necessary for him to have a CT angiogram, the most critical step before a CT angiogram is control of his blood pressure and pain. Anti-impulse therapy with labetalol infusion and opiate analgesia should proceed with a computerised tomography angiogram when this diagnosis is highly suspected.

Q3. Option B – He should start on an antiplatelet agent and a statin and be advised to stop smoking. He should have a review of his diabetes management and see a podiatrist for foot care. No imaging is necessary, and he is advised to attend a supervised exercise programme.

Claudication is a lifestyle-limiting disease and not limb-threatening. This question highlights a patient who does not appear to have lifestyle-limiting claudication whilst at the same time he has many risk factors that require management. At this stage, it would be appropriate to manage him without surgical or radiological intervention, and therefore, there is no indication for any imaging at this stage such as a CT angiogram or even an arterial duplex scan. He clearly has peripheral vascular disease related to atherosclerosis with likely aorto-iliac occlusive disease. He requires antiplatelet therapy and statins for secondary cardiovascular protection. He requires his other risk factors to be managed including smoking and diabetes. There is good evidence that a supervised exercise programme can improve his walking distance and quality of life.

Q4. Option A – Give 5,000 u bolus of unfractionated heparin, arrange an immediate arterial duplex scan and take her to the theatre to perform a brachial embolectomy under local anaesthesia.

This patient presents with a typical history of an embolus causing acute upper limb ischaemia. The management involves giving unfractionated heparin as soon as the diagnosis is suspected, and arterial duplex ultrasonography can be very helpful and rapidly performed to aid in diagnosis. A simple brachial embolectomy can be performed under a local anaesthetic, and in this patient, there is no indication to consider fasciotomy from the history provided. The management of atrial fibrillation will be necessary, but cardioversion would risk further embolisation when performed during the same admission. Thrombolysis would not be appropriate in this patient as it takes a long period of time to successfully lyse the clot and it would incur unnecessary risk to the patient. The patient will need to be anticoagulated after surgery and the source of the embolus be investigated.

Q5. Option D – Recommend that she is admitted from the clinic under vascular surgeons with the view to the treatment of her 4.9 cm infra-renal AAA.

This patient has a symptomatic AAA which in itself is an indication for treatment despite the fact that the aneurysm measures less than 5.5 cm in diameter. A tender aneurysm requires urgent admission and issues and should be considered to be a contained rupture until proven otherwise. An urgent computerised tomography angiogram should be performed, and the patient should be admitted under the care of the vascular surgeons. Even if no signs of any rupture or present on the computerised tomography scan, this aneurysm should be treated during the same admission.

Q6. Option A – Start the patient on an antiplatelet agent and statin. Repeat carotid duplex scan at a specialised vascular centre, and if findings are similar, arrange for urgent left carotid endarterectomy within 2 weeks of his initial symptoms.

This patient has suffered a TIA affecting the left cerebral hemisphere. Therefore, he has 90% right internal carotid artery stenosis and he is asymptomatic. He requires antiplatelet therapy and initiation of statin. This patient should be referred from a TIA clinic directly to a basket seen where it is standard practice to repeat a carotid duplex scan in the specialised centre. Symptomatic carotid stenosis above 50% is an indication of carotid surgery. If there is doubt in the findings of the carotid duplex scan, then a computerised tomography angiogram can be helpful. It is unusual to perform a carotid angiogram for diagnostic purposes, and it is not standard practice to start this sort of patient on a heparin infusion. Current guidelines would consider this patient for carotid endarterectomy on an urgent basis and insert within 2 weeks of the symptoms to avoid the TIA or stroke.

Q7. Option D – Arrange an arterial duplex of the coeliac, superior and inferior mesenteric arteries to assess for any significant stenoses.

This patient presents with a typical history suggestive of mesenteric angina. However, it is important to rule out nonvascular causes of abdominal pain and weight loss first. The CT scan which was performed without contrast raises the suspicion of mesenteric artery disease because of the presence of aortic and mesenteric calcification. A diagnosis of mesenteric angina would be supported by a fasting and post-prandial mesenteric arterial duplex scan. Whilst a CT scan with contrast in the mesenteric phase would be very useful, it may result in significant nephrotoxicity. Similarly, an invasive procedure such as a diagnostic catheter angiogram is an unnecessary risk for diagnosis alone.

Q8. Option D – Anticoagulation should be commenced immediately and a venous duplex scan performed to establish if she has an axillary and subclavian vein thrombosis.

This is a typical story of effort thrombosis or Paget Schoettler's syndrome. An urgent venous duplex scan will diagnose an axillary and or subclavian vein thrombosis quickly. There is no need to perform a venogram or MRI scan to be able to get a diagnosis. Anticoagulation is mandatory on suspicion of axillary vein thrombosis as a small number of these will result in a pulmonary embolus. It is standard practice to offer the patient the option of catheter-directed thrombolysis with or without mechanical thrombectomy and to decompress the thoracic outlet. However, some patients are best treated simply by anticoagulation and conservative management alone.

Q9. Option A – The patient should have a computerised tomography scan with arterial phase contrast and undergo cardiovascular risk assessment prior to being offered open surgery for his large AAA.

This patient has met the indication for the repair of his AAA. He is a young relatively fit man and is likely to be best suited for open repair rather than endovascular stent graft because of its length to his durability. He will require a computerised tomography angiogram to evaluate his AAA better prior to undergoing surgery. Cardiovascular risk stratification is often performed as a cardiopulmonary exercise test (CPET) as a static echocardiogram does not help risk stratification patients.

Q10. Option D – A venous duplex scan should be performed to establish the extent of superficial thrombophlebitis, and she should be recommended to wear class 2 graduated above-knee compression stockings and take nonsteroidal anti-inflammatory drugs (NSAIDs). Once superficial thrombophlebitis has settled down, she should be considered for treatment of her superficial venous insufficiency.

One of the complications of varicose veins is superficial thrombophlebitis. This is an indication for treatment of the underlying superficial venous insufficiency. However, treatment is best performed when the inflammatory phase is settled. Initial management includes graduated compression stockings and nonsteroidal anti-inflammatory drugs (NSAIDs). The patient should be well hydrated and remain active and avoid prolonged bed rest. There is no indication of formal anticoagulation in most cases of superficial thrombophlebitis. However, if there is concern that a deep vein thrombosis may be present, hold the phlebitis extensions close to the sapheno-femoral or saphenopopliteal junctions, and then there may be a role for formal anticoagulation. The diagnosis is made on venous duplex ultrasound imaging and does not require a venogram.

Q11. Option E – The patient should be reassessed with ABPI being measured and a biopsy of the edge of the ulcer being performed. A venous duplex scan would be recommended prior to considering any form of superficial venous treatment.

This patient has a venous leg ulcer that has not healed with traditional therapy and therefore another aetiology should be considered. It is important that arterial insufficiency is considered. An ABPI of greater than 0.8 is required to allow for leg-graduated compression bandaging. A squamous cell cancer change in the ulcer should also be considered particularly if the edges of the ulcer are irregular and suspicious. A biopsy of the edge of the ulcer should be performed in that situation. Superficial venous treatment by means of endovenous ablation therapy or surgery is proven to reduce the frequency of recurrence of venous leg ulcers but does not expedite healing rates. A venous duplex scan is mandatory before considering treatment of superficial venous insufficiency in a patient with venous leg ulcers to confirm the status of the deep veins.

Q12. Option E – Ultrasound-guided compression of the false aneurysm for at least 20 minutes should be attempted, and if this fails to thrombose the false aneurysm, then ultrasound-guided thrombin injection should be performed.

A pseudoaneurysm or false aneurysm is a recognised complication of an arterial puncture. Pseudoaneurysms after cardiac catheterisation are often treated by ultrasound-guided compression or ultrasound-guided thrombin injection. In combination, these treatments have at least a 90% success rate. If surgical repair is required, it usually only requires direct closure of the hole in the artery and does not require ligation and interposition grafting. This is unlike the situation with IV drug users who develop a false aneurysm. In these patients, the hole in the artery is usually large and infected and cannot be managed by ultrasound-guided compression or thrombin injection. Whilst a covered stent graft is an option for treating pseudoaneurysms, it is only really considered in patients not fit for surgery.

Q13. Option D – Aorto-uni-iliac EVAR and right-to left femoro-femoral crossover bypass.

This patient has critical limb ischaemia as well as an AAA with left iliac artery thrombosis. Whilst the aneurysm has not reached the threshold for intervention, it is nonetheless necessary to treat this at the same time as improving the flow to his left leg. A thrombectomy of the left iliac artery alone would not be sufficient because there is a large volume of thrombus within the AAA that is likely to cause further problems in the future with emboli or thrombosis of the iliac vessels. It is not appropriate to use a bifurcated endovascular this aneurysm stent graft given the left iliac occlusion, but an aorto-uni-iliac EVAR with a right-to-left femoro-femoro crossover graft will treat both the AAA as well as the left leg critical limb ischaemia.

Q14. Option B – Venous duplex scan, compression bandage dressing and endovenous ablation for superficial varicosities only if deep veins are patent.

Q15. Option C – Oral anticoagulation for 6 months and decompression of the TOS only if duplex scan demonstrated venous recanalisation.

Q16. Option B – Consider fasciotomy if the compartment pressure is 35 mmHg or higher.

Q17. Option D – Left carotid endarterectomy CEA is less beneficial after 6 weeks post-event and the best medical therapy is enough to manage this lady.

Q18. Option D – CT scan to confirm ruptured AAA.

Q19. Option A – Unilateral extensive iliofemoral DVT.

Q20. Option D – Left aorto-femoral bypass.

Index

Note: **Bold** page numbers refer to tables and *italic* page numbers refer to figures.